DESCRIBING DEATH IN AMERICA
What We Need to Know

June R. Lunney, Kathleen M. Foley, Thomas J. Smith, and
Hellen Gelband, *Editors*

National Cancer Policy Board
and
Division of Earth and Life Studies

INSTITUTE OF MEDICINE
NATIONAL RESEARCH COUNCIL
OF THE NATIONAL ACADEMIES

THE NATIONAL ACADEMIES PRESS
Washington, D.C.
www.nap.edu

THE NATIONAL ACADEMIES PRESS • 500 Fifth Street, N.W. • Washington, DC 20001

NOTICE: The project that is the subject of this report was approved by the Governing Board of the National Research Council, whose members are drawn from the councils of the National Academy of Sciences, the National Academy of Engineering, and the Institute of Medicine. The members of the committee responsible for the report were chosen for their special competences and with regard for appropriate balance.

Support for this project was provided by the National Cancer Institute, the Centers for Disease and Prevention, and the American Cancer Society. The views presented in this report are those of the National Cancer Policy Board and are not necessarily those of the funding agencies.

Library of Congress Cataloging-in-Publication Data

Describing death in America : what we need to know / Kathleen M. Foley
... [et al.], editors ; National Cancer Policy Board, Institute of
Medicine, and Division on Earth and Life Studies, National Research
Council.
   p. ; cm.
Includes bibliographical references.
 ISBN 0-309-08725-2 (pbk.)
 1. Terminal care—United States. 2. Cancer—Palliative
treatment—United States.
 [DNLM: 1. Terminal Care—United States. 2. Data Collection—United
States. 3. Mortality—United States. 4. Quality Assurance, Health
Care—United States. 5. Quality of Life—United States. 6. Terminally
Ill—psychology—United States. WB 310 D449 2003] I. Foley, Kathleen
M., 1944- II. National Cancer Policy Board (U.S.) III. National Research
Council (U.S.). Division on Earth and Life Studies.
 R726.8.D475 2003
 616.99′4029—dc21

2003000881

Additional copies of this report are available for sale from the National Academies Press, 500 Fifth Street, N.W., Lockbox 285, Washington, DC 20055; call (800) 624-6242 or (202) 334-3313 (in the Washington metropolitan area); Internet, http://www.nap.edu.

For more information about the Institute of Medicine, visit the IOM home page at: **www.iom.edu.**

THE NATIONAL ACADEMIES
Advisers to the Nation on Science, Engineering, and Medicine

The **National Academy of Sciences** is a private, nonprofit, self-perpetuating society of distinguished scholars engaged in scientific and engineering research, dedicated to the furtherance of science and technology and to their use for the general welfare. Upon the authority of the charter granted to it by the Congress in 1863, the Academy has a mandate that requires it to advise the federal government on scientific and technical matters. Dr. Bruce M. Alberts is president of the National Academy of Sciences.

The **National Academy of Engineering** was established in 1964, under the charter of the National Academy of Sciences, as a parallel organization of outstanding engineers. It is autonomous in its administration and in the selection of its members, sharing with the National Academy of Sciences the responsibility for advising the federal government. The National Academy of Engineering also sponsors engineering programs aimed at meeting national needs, encourages education and research, and recognizes the superior achievements of engineers. Dr. Wm. A. Wulf is president of the National Academy of Engineering.

The **Institute of Medicine** was established in 1970 by the National Academy of Sciences to secure the services of eminent members of appropriate professions in the examination of policy matters pertaining to the health of the public. The Institute acts under the responsibility given to the National Academy of Sciences by its congressional charter to be an adviser to the federal government and, upon its own initiative, to identify issues of medical care, research, and education. Dr. Harvey V. Fineberg is president of the Institute of Medicine.

The **National Research Council** was organized by the National Academy of Sciences in 1916 to associate the broad community of science and technology with the Academy's purposes of furthering knowledge and advising the federal government. Functioning in accordance with general policies determined by the Academy, the Council has become the principal operating agency of both the National Academy of Sciences and the National Academy of Engineering in providing services to the government, the public, and the scientific and engineering communities. The Council is administered jointly by both Academies and the Institute of Medicine. Dr. Bruce M. Alberts and Dr. Wm. A. Wulf are chair and vice chair, respectively, of the National Research Council.

www.national-academies.org

Reviewers

This report has been reviewed in draft form by individuals chosen for their diverse perspectives and technical expertise, in accordance with procedures approved by the NRC's Report Review Committee. The purpose of this independent review is to provide candid and critical comments that will assist the institution in making its published report as sound as possible and to ensure that the report meets institutional standards for objectivity, evidence, and responsiveness to the study charge. The review comments and draft manuscript remain confidential to protect the integrity of the deliberative process. We wish to thank the following individuals for their review of this report:

Nicholas Christakis, Harvard University
Betty Ferrell, City of Hope National Medical Center
Joanne M. Hilden, The Cleveland Clinic
Vincent Mor, Providence, Rhode Island
James A. Tulsky, VA Medical Center, Durham, North Carolina
Beth Virnig, University of Minnesota

Although the reviewers listed above have provided many constructive comments and suggestions, they were not asked to endorse the conclusions or recommendations nor did they see the final draft of the report before its release. The review of this report was overseen by Samuel H. Preston, University of Pennsylvania and George E. Thibault, Partners HealthCare System, Inc. Appointed by the National Research Council and Institute of Medicine, they were responsible for making certain that an independent examination of this report was carried out in accordance with institutional procedures and that all review comments were carefully considered. Responsibility for the final content of this report rests entirely with the authoring committee and the institution.

Acronyms and Abbreviations

AHEAD   Asset and Health Dynamics Among the Oldest Old Study
CMS   Centers for Medicare and Medicaid Services
DHHS   Department of Health and Human Services
DMIS   Defense Medical Information System
FERRET   Federal Electronic Research and Review Extraction Tool
GAO   General Accounting Office
HC   Household Component
HEDIS   Health Plan Employer Data and Information Set
HRS   Health and Retirement Study
IC   Insurance Component
IOM   Institute of Medicine
JCAHO   Joint Commission on the Accreditation of Healthcare Organizations
LSOA   Longitudinal Study of Aging
MCBS   Medicare Current Beneficiary Survey
MDS   Nursing Home Minimum Data Set
MedPAC   Medicare Payment Advisory Commission
MPC   Medical Provider Component
NCQA   National Committee for Quality Assurance
NHC   Nursing Home Component
NIH   National Institutes of Health
NIS   Nationwide Inpatient Sample
NLTCS   National Long-Term Care Surveys

NMES   National Medical Care Expenditure Survey
NMFS   National Mortality Followback Survey
OASIS   Outcome and Assessment Information Set
PSID   Panel Study of Income Dynamics
PTF   Patient Treatment File
RAI   Resident Assessment Instrument
SASD   State Ambulatory Surgery Databases
SEER   Surveillance, Epidemiology, and End Results Program
SID   State Inpatient Databases
SOA   Supplement on Aging
SOAII   Second Supplement on Aging

Contents

DESCRIBING DEATH IN AMERICA

Executive Summary

In the United States today, we know with reasonable certainty what people die from, how old they are when they die, and some other key pieces of information. Trends over time in these vital statistics, and associated research on factors that tend to increase or decrease the risk of death, have laid the foundation for strategies to improve public health and avoid premature deaths. But death does come—to about 2.4 million each year. Although death is largely a phenomenon of old age, deaths among younger people are significant, adding up to half a million infants, children and young adults. We have only begun to pay attention to the circumstances in which chronically ill people approach death and experience the dying process. We know relatively little about the quality, appropriateness, or costs of care they receive, or the burden on caregivers and survivors. Even less is known about deaths of young people than about deaths among middle-aged and elderly people (Seeman et al., 1989).

"Quality of care" is a subjective concept, of course, but various groups have begun to define minimum standards that can be agreed upon, as well as ideals that can be held as goals. Quality of care is not an end in itself, either for the temporarily or the fatally ill. It is one contributor to "quality of life," regardless of the amount of time left to a life. In this report, we are concerned about describing both "quality of care" and "quality of life" near the end of life. They are distinct qualities and require different types of measurements, related either to the process and outcomes of care, in the former case, or the perceptions of the dying and those around them, in the latter.

1

The National Cancer Policy Board concluded in its July 2001 report, *Improving Palliative Care for Cancer* (IOM, 2001), that there is currently insufficient information to assess or improve the quality of care provided to those who die from cancer in the United States. The Board noted that we have little understanding of the particular dying experiences of most patients with cancer—where they die, who cares for them as they are dying, what the quality of such care is, whether care guidelines are being followed, and whether these things are changing over time. This lack of information hampers our ability to develop a clear policy agenda and will, in the future, impede monitoring trends to determine whether interventions are having their intended effects of improving the quality of life for individuals at the end of life.

Knowing how well we are doing or whether things are getting better in end-of-life care requires some routinely collected information. It may be possible to make better use of data already being collected (including those collected for other purposes), but it also may be desirable or necessary to gather new types of data. The Board, therefore, decided to undertake an assessment of the information potential of current data sources to assess quality of life and quality of care at the end of life. Recognizing that the issue existed not only for deaths from cancer, but for all deaths, this report was undertaken in collaboration with the Board on Health Sciences Policy in this project that looks at deaths from all causes and at all ages, including childhood.

This report reviews the sources of information currently available that shed light on the quality of care and quality of life at the end of life. It has uncovered wide gaps between what we would like to know and what is actually known or knowable, if existing national-level data were fully explored and analyzed. The scope of the report is limited to examining large-scale data collection through vital statistics, ongoing national surveys, administrative data from the Medicare program, and some large periodic surveys. Data from these sources, if fully exploited, can provide a framework—a skeleton—for the complete story, which can be told only through the many types of hypothesis-driven epidemiologic and health services studies that are critical to filling in the details of quality of care and quality of life of real people who are dying. Often, it is the national-level data collection efforts described in this report that are used to generate hypotheses to be tested in more focused studies. And while this report delves into the types of data needed, it does not include an analysis of current funding levels, or of the funds that would be needed to carry out the recommendations. That said, however, there is a clear theme of striving for the best use of existing data, and where changes are required—either modifications of existing systems or new efforts—proposing how to accomplish them with the fewest perturbations.

WHY WE NEED TO KNOW

There are various reasons for wanting to find out more about the circumstances of people's lives as they are approaching death. The focus of this report and its recommendations is on the quality of care and quality of life during the period leading up to death for people with progressive disease. The rationale becomes clear when viewed as a logical next report in relation to its immediate predecessor, *Improving Palliative Care for Cancer* (IOM, 2001), and the 1997 Institute of Medicine (IOM) report *Approaching Death: Improving Care at the End of Life.* The care of individuals who are approaching death is an integral and important part of health care (IOM, 1997). Furthermore, people who are nearing the end of life should be able to expect and achieve a decent or good death—one that is free from avoidable distress and suffering for patients, families, and caregivers; in general accord with patients' and families' wishes; and reasonably consistent with clinical, cultural, and ethical standards (IOM, 1997). We know from studies and from anecdotal information that for too many people, this expectation is not being met. But if we want to know how we're doing as a nation, we must gather information systematically and regularly, in a way that will allow comparisons across different segments of society and over time.

The experience of dying today is typically very different from what it was 100 years ago. Death at home in the care of the family has been replaced in most instances by a technological, professional, and institutional treatment of dying (IOM, 1997). A theme of the 1997 *Approaching Death* report was that a significant number of people experience needless suffering and distress at the end of life. The suffering and distress is caused in some cases when caregivers provide care that is clinically inappropriate or not wanted by the patient; in other cases, it results when caregivers underuse effective treatments to relieve pain or other physical or psychological symptoms (IOM, 1997). As a consequence, many Americans "have come both to fear a technologically overtreated and protracted death and to dread the prospect of abandonment and untreated physical and emotional distress" (IOM, 1997).

In order to improve the quality of life and quality of care for people at the end of life, it will be necessary to develop, validate, and benchmark measures of quality for end-of-life care. As W. Edwards Deming stated, "If you don't measure it, you can't improve it." Measures of the quality of life and care of dying patients are needed for the purposes of (1) *public accountability* (i.e., allowing policymakers, patients, families, and the public to hold organizations and individuals accountable for the quality of the care they provide to dying patients); (2) *internal quality improvement efforts* by clinicians and others directly responsible for end-of-life care to evaluate and improve what they are doing on a continuing basis; and (3) further *research* on the effects of different clinical, organizational, and financing options for end-of-life care and on the effectiveness of alternative strategies for improving care and outcomes for patients and their families (IOM, 1997; Teno, 2001).

At this point, the understanding of what it means to live well while dying and how to measure the quality of dying remains at an early stage (IOM, 1997; Teno, 2001). Basic descriptions of the dying experience and the care given to people who are dying are lacking (Teno, 2001). Clinical guidelines to help physicians, nurses, and other health professionals manage life-threatening illnesses are generally silent on the topic of managing the end stage of the disease (IOM, 2001; Teno, 2001). The field of palliative care focuses on the prevention and relief of suffering through the final stages of an illness and attends closely to the emotional, spiritual, and practical needs of patients and those close to them, but there are no quality indicators in national use that deal specifically with the quality of palliative care provided to patients with life-threatening and incurable illnesses (Teno, 2001).

Strengthening accountability for dying patients' quality of life and care will require better data and tools for evaluating outcomes important to patients and families (IOM, 1997). Patient preferences and satisfaction are important at every stage of treatment, but they have particular significance in the care of patients with life-threatening and incurable illnesses (Teno, 2001). One category of outcomes in dying patients for which there is particularly strong normative and empirical evidence to support quality measures is pain management (Teno, 2001). In 1997, the IOM reported on the American Geriatrics Society suggestions for other domains of quality of care for dying patients, among them physical and emotional symptoms, support of functioning and autonomy, advance care planning, aggressive care near death, patient and family satisfaction, and global quality of life (IOM, 1997). Only after satisfactory measures in end-of-life quality domains such as these are developed and evaluated in demonstration programs will it be possible to develop and apply standards of accountability for end-of-life care. All of this begins with knowing something about how people across the country are dying now.

WHAT WE NEED TO KNOW

The effort to better understand and to improve the care received by those at the end of life will require better information about dying—not just about the demographic characteristics and health conditions of those who die, but also about their quality of life as they cope with declining health, the quality of their death, and the quality of the health care provided to them during this time. Nationally representative surveys, disease registries, health care billing data and vital statistics are among the possible sources of this information. To date, the focus of most analyses of these data has been on factors contributing to death, rather than on the experience of dying. To better understand dying, a very different set of topics would be of interest. These might include characteristics of the site of death, symptoms and quality of life in the last year of life for patients and their families, patient preferences for and continuity of care in the last year of life, and family burden (physical, psychological, practical, and financial).

Designating a period of time as "the end of life" is a difficult but necessary first step. The conceptual model of a "terminal illness" has driven most current public policy about dying, though dying is not so easily predictable for most Americans. Death more frequently occurs during an exacerbation of an otherwise chronic illness or from a complication associated with a very long slow decline in old age (Lunney et al., 2001). In this report, the end of life is defined very broadly, to include the period during which an individual copes with declining health from an ultimately terminal illness, from a serious though perhaps chronic illness, or from the frailties associated with advanced age—even if death is not clearly imminent.

Public discussions and focus group research have helped us to understand what the American public values in the care of the dying (Steinhauser et al., 2000a, b; Teno et al., 2001). Professional societies and experts in palliative and end-of-life care have also developed frameworks that describe the concerns of people who are dying, and the roles of professionals, family members, and society at large in meeting their needs. The various frameworks use different terminology, and may split into different components, but basically, they all include:

- The management of symptoms;
- Spiritual and personal growth;
- A familiar setting, surrounded by loved ones;
- Understandable information to guide decision making and planning;
- Confidence that one will not be a financial, emotional, or physical burden to family members; and
- The right of self-determination and control of treatment choices.

These frameworks and the "domains" they include lead directly to specific questions that must be answered to assess and monitor how well needs are being met. We have taken the elements in the various models and developed a set of questions that would capture the information

TABLE ES-1 Questions to Assess and Monitor How Well Individuals'
End-of-Life Needs Are Being Met

1. Where are people dying and how much of the end of their lives is spent in those settings?

2. Who is providing care for them as they die? Do institutional settings support family presence at the end of life?

3. Are physical and psychological symptoms being identified and treated (including but not limited to pain)?

4. What proportion of people experience impaired cognitive function before death, to what degree, and for what period of time?

5. What proportion of people experience physical disability or social isolation before death, to what degree, and for what period of time?

6. How do patients and loved ones perceive their quality of life at various time points prior to death?

7. Are patients and loved ones achieving a sense of life closure in their relationships and spiritually?

8. Are patients and loved ones involved in decision making about treatment and care options?

9. Are patients and loved ones receiving timely and adequate information on which to base informed decisions?

10. Are patients and loved ones receiving supportive services from chaplains, therapists, health aides, and other providers?

11. Are family physical, emotional,   and financial resources being heavily depleted by the care of a dying family member?

12. Are loved ones supported through the grieving process?

needed to fill in important blanks (see Table ES-1). These questions are used later to query the data sets described, to determine how well each question is covered (summarized in Table ES-2, and more fully discussed in Chapter 3).

SOURCES OF DATA

Very few efforts to gather data specifically to illuminate the issues surrounding dying and the end of life have been made, but data are routinely collected for other purposes that can fill some of the needs. In some cases, data simply must be extracted and analyzed to prove useful, and in other cases, changes in what is collected routinely could greatly improve the usefulness of various data sources for these purposes. Chapter 3 of this report describes large datasets, including both ongoing and periodic or one-time surveys, that contain some relevant elements. These range from the death certificate, which is completed for every person who dies in the United States and aggregated in national mortality reporting, to billing records for the Medicare program, to regular or episodic surveys of representative samples of individuals in the general population (e.g., the continuous National Health Interview Survey and the now continuous, but formerly episodic National Health and Nutrition Examination Survey, both conducted by the National Center for Health Statistics). Mortality "followback" surveys, in which proxy respondents (usually surviving spouses or other family members) are interviewed to gather information about people who died in a given year, have great potential to answer directly some of the questions identified, but the last one took place in 1993 and no new followback surveys are planned (but see Recommendations, below).

In Chapter 3, the large-scale data sources with information relevant to end-of-life concerns are described and reviewed for the useful elements they contain. This information is summarized in Table ES-2 and provides the background against which recommendations described below have been developed. Methodological issues involved in studying the quality of life and care at the end of life are described in Chapter 4.

CONCLUSIONS AND RECOMMENDATIONS

The final chapter of the report summarizes conclusions and presents the Institute of Medicine's recommendations. It notes that a better description of how Americans of all ages currently die and the impact on their families is much needed and must be followed by continuing efforts to track changes over time. Both the quality of dying and the quality of the health care provided at the end of life should be addressed.

The IOM's recommendations, summarized below, address supporting the use of existing data systems, improving the usefulness of existing data systems, and undertaking new data collection efforts to learn about the quality of life and care at the end of life.

Recommendation #1:
Support Researchers' Use of Existing Data Systems

Agencies should promote research that uses existing data resources to describe aspects of the quality of life and quality of care at the end of life, by publicizing their availability and providing funding for analysis.

TABLE ES-2 Types of Data Available from Datasets That Contain Individual-Level Information

Data type		Number of deaths year[s]	Cause of death	Comorbidities	Pain or other physical symptoms
C2	AHEAD	1,900 (1993-98)		✓	✓
C2	LSOA I & II	I: 2,900 (1984-90) II: 1,900 (1994-2000)	✓	✓	
C1	MCBS	700/yr		✓	
B	MDS			✓	✓
B	Medicare claims	1.7 million (2000)		✓	
C1	MEPS	NA[2]		✓	✓
A	Death Certificates (NDI)	2.4 M (2000)	✓		
C1	NHANES	50/yr estimate		✓	✓
C2	NHEFS	1,400 (1987-92)[1]	✓	✓	✓
C2	NHHCS	~5,000 (2000)		✓	
C1	NHIS	55,000 (1986-94)		✓	✓
C2	NLTCS	17,000 (1982-86)		✓	
C2	NMFS	23,000 (1993)	✓	✓	
C1	NNHS	~1,600 (1999)		✓	
B	OASIS			✓	✓
C1	PSID	4,300 (thru 1999)		✓	

Physical function	Psychological symptoms	QoL	Cognition	Site of death	Lived with	Social support
✓	✓	✓	✓		✓	✓
✓				✓	✓	✓
✓			✓		✓	✓
✓	✓		✓		✓	✓
✓	✓		✓		✓	
				✓		
✓			✓		✓	
✓				✓	✓	
✓					✓	
✓	✓		✓		✓	
✓	✓		✓		✓	✓
✓			✓	✓	✓	
✓					✓	
✓	✓		✓		✓	
✓					✓	

TABLE ES-2 Continued

Data type		Family care	Out of pocket expenses	Bereavement	ADS
C2	AHEAD	✓	✓		✓
C2	LSOA I & II	✓			✓
C1	MCBS		✓		
B	MDS		✓		✓
B	Medicare claims				
C1	MEPS	✓	✓		
A	Death Certificates (NDI)				
C1	NHANES				
C2	NHEFS				
C2	NHHCS	✓	✓		
C1	NHIS		✓		
C2	NLTCS	✓	✓		✓
C2	NMFS	✓	✓		✓
C1	NNHS		✓		
B	OASIS	✓			
C1	PSID	✓			

KEY: First Column: A = Vital statistics; B = Administrative data; C = Research sample (C1 = continuous or regular sample; C2 = not continuous or regularly occurring sample); AHEAD—Asset and Health Dynamics Among the Oldest Old; LSOA—Longitudinal Survey of Aging; MCBS—Medicare Current Beneficiary Survey; MDS—nursing home Minimum Data Set; MEPS—Medicare Expenditure Panel Survey; NDI—National Death Index; NHANES—National Health and Nutrition Examination Survey; NHEFS—NHANES I Epidemiologic Followup Survey; NHHCS—National Home and Hospice Care Survey; NHIS—National Health Interview Survey; NLTCS—National

Decision making	Satisfaction	Support	Use of services	Quality	Provider
			✓		
			✓		
	✓	✓	✓	✓	
		✓	✓		
			✓		✓
	✓	✓	✓	✓	✓
			✓		
			✓		
		✓	✓		
			✓	✓	
		✓	✓		
✓		✓	✓	✓	
		✓			✓
		✓	✓		✓
			✓		

Long-Term Care Survey; NMFS—National Mortality Followback Survey; NNHS—National Nursing Home Survey; OASIS—Outcome and Assessment Information Set; PSID—Panel Study of Income Dynamics.

[1]Deaths during 5-year follow-up period total 20-year follow-up (1971-1992).
[2]MEPS data will be linked to the NDI when a large enough number of deaths have occurred. It is currently too early for this.

A great deal of information is recorded, for a variety of purposes, that could describe aspects of quality of life and quality of care at the end of life. It is probably not surprising that Medicare claims and other data collected for purposes other than measuring quality at the end of life are not always used to their fullest for measuring quality, given that their primary purpose is purely administrative. In addition, the full potential value of many surveys and studies of health and well-being in characterizing quality of life and care at the end of life is not realized because data are analyzed only to answer some questions but not others. The reasons for this vary, but include a general lack of funding support for further data analysis, the fact that researchers are unaware of the data resource, and in some cases, the relatively new ability to link data from different sources to facilitate meaningful answers to important questions.

Currently, little support is available to researchers to make use of existing data resources in describing aspects of the quality of life and and the care provided to individuals who are dying. Research-funding agencies should provide support for using existing data resources for this purpose. Some examples of the types of studies that could be conducted with modest funding include:

- Making use of existing longitudinal surveys to examine the health trajectories of those who die in order to learn more about the role of suffering, disability, and chronic illnesses at the end of life.
- Studying patterns of costs and utilization in the years before death to more fully describe the use of home care, hospice care, in-home privately paid help, and informal care.
- Studying the number of care transitions in the last year of life, both in terms of settings and of providers.
- Comparing data from multiple settings with regard to the rates of pain and other symptom assessment, and use of opioids and other symptom-relieving interventions.
- Developing valid indicators of variables and constructs that are important to good end-of-life care. This is an important but slow process—and one that needs to be attended to immediately.
- Examining individual and institutional factors that influence racial and geographic variations in patterns of end-of-life care.

Recommendation #2:
Improve the Usefulness of Existing Data Systems

Government and private organizations should institute training initiatives and make incremental changes to surveys to improve the

usefulness of currently collected data in describing aspects of quality of life and quality of care at the end of life.

Training for researchers and incremental changes to surveys would be relatively inexpensive ways to improve the usefulness of currently collected data in describing aspects of quality of life and quality of care at the end of life.

Training for Researchers

More funding for analysis and better publicity about data sources will improve the use of existing information up to a point, but beyond that, researchers may need training in specific datasets or enhancement of skills to be able to understand the possibilities of existing information collection. Focused training opportunities, limited in scope, can open the way for much better use of what data currently exist. Specific recommendations for training of researchers are as follows:

• Government agencies that sponsor data collection should sponsor a series of training initiatives to open dialogues among researchers and health care workers to increase the reliability and validity of ongoing data collections. These should emphasize:

  • Training professionals in various disciplines in the use of data sources.
  • Training existing palliative care researchers to incorporate research questions in their studies, which would utilize existing data bases.
  • Promoting existing health service researchers with expertise in these databases to collaborate with palliative care researchers.

Improving the Quality of Data Recorded

• Professional organizations should promote increased standardization of language through open dialogue about terms that now have diverse meanings, e.g., hospice care, palliative care, and end of life.
• In settings where physicians complete death certificates regularly, institute training and quality control measures.
• The federal government should mandate that institutions and organizations providing care (hospitals, nursing homes, home health agencies, outpatient settings) conduct ongoing quality improvement efforts, including training in recording required data.

Incremental Changes to Ongoing Data Collection Efforts

The information content for studying end-of-life issues can be enhanced in specific surveys by relatively minor changes. The following improvements, modifications, or supplements to ongoing data collection efforts would be relatively inexpensive ways to build upon existing efforts:

- Sponsors of longitudinal health surveys should insist on the routine use of "exit" surveys to capture information from the next-of-kin of participants who die between survey rounds. These supplemental surveys not only enhance the existing survey by covering a more inclusive range of outcomes but can provide rich data about end-of-life issues at relatively low cost.
- Improvements to the information infrastructure, such as nationwide electronic reporting of death certificates, should be made to facilitate more timely collection and analysis of vital information.
- Sampling frames for current surveys should be carefully reviewed for adequacy both in terms of contemporary housing arrangements and changing health care organizational structures.
- Survey questions regarding health care utilization should include probes that capture need for and use of the full range of supportive services.
- Mechanisms should be put in place for continuous refinement of large ongoing surveys, using input from a wide variety of sources. Web-based opportunities to e-mail questions and suggestions would facilitate this exchange.
- The Centers for Medicare and Medicaid Services (CMS)—formerly known as the Health Care Financing Administration—should consider minor increases in the data elements recorded on Medicare claims under the hospice benefit. This topic should be addressed by the Medicare Payment Advisory Commission (MedPAC), a Congressionally-mandated organization that advises CMS on the Medicare system. Ongoing efforts should be directed towards facilitating links among key types of data collection, especially between surveys and health care utilization records.

Recommendation #3:
A New National Mortality Followback Survey

The federal government should undertake a new National Mortality Followback Survey to enhance the accuracy and richness of data collection related to quality of life and care at the end of life.

A new National Mortality Followback Survey program of regular, periodic surveys that gather comparable data over time, should be initiated. The new NMFS would be a collaborative effort between the National Center for Health Statistics (which would carry out the survey), the National Institutes of Health (NIH), and the Agency for Healthcare Research and Quality (the latter organizations would sponsor the survey). As the lead institute for end-of-life research at the NIH, the National Institute of Nursing Research could take a major role in supporting a National Mortality Followback Survey and determining content, with collaboration from other NIH institutes (in particular, the National Institute on Aging, but possibly including some of the disease-oriented institutes), and the Agency for Healthcare Research and Quality. Three specific aims should be considered for future National Mortality Followback Surveys. First, a major focus should be on determining the extent of morbidity experienced at the end of life, to aid the long-range goal of reducing unnecessary morbidity. Second, deaths among children should be over-sampled in order to yield information specific to this understudied group. And third, minority populations should be over-sampled to improve understanding of ethnic and racial differences in the experience of death and dying in the United States.

I

Introduction and Overview

The National Cancer Policy Board concluded in its July 2001 report, *Improving Palliative Care for Cancer* (IOM, 2001), that there is currently insufficient information to assess the quality of care provided to those who die from cancer in the United States. The Board noted that we have little understanding of the particular dying experiences of most patients with cancer—where they die, who cares for them as they are dying, what the quality of such care is, whether relevant guidelines are being followed, and whether these things are changing over time. This lack of information hampers our ability to develop a clear policy agenda and will, in the future, impede monitoring trends to determine whether interventions are having their intended effects of improving the quality of life and care for individuals at the end of life.

"Quality of care" is a subjective concept, of course, but various groups have begun to define some minimum standards that can be agreed upon, as well as ideals to be considered. Quality of care is not an end in itself, either for the temporarily or the fatally ill. It is one factor that can contribute to "quality of life," regardless of the amount of time left to that life. In this report, we are concerned about describing both "quality of care" and "quality of life" near the end of life. They are distinct qualities and require different types of measurements, related either to the process and outcomes of care, in the former case, or the perceptions of the dying and those around them, in the latter.

Knowing how well we are doing or whether things are getting better in end-of-life care requires some routinely collected information. It may be possible to make better use of data already being collected (including those collected for other purposes), but it also may be desirable or necessary to gather new types of data. The Board, therefore, decided to undertake an assessment of the information potential of current data sources to assess quality of life and quality of care at the end of life. Recognizing that the issue existed not only for deaths from cancer, but for all deaths, this report was undertaken in collaboration with the Board on Health Sciences Policy in this project that looks at deaths from all causes and at all ages, including childhood.

BACKGROUND ON END-OF-LIFE ISSUES

The National Cancer Policy Board was established in March 1997 at the Institute of Medicine (IOM) and National Research Council to address issues that arise in the prevention, control, diagnosis, treatment, and palliation of cancer. In April 1999, the National Cancer Policy Board released a report, *Ensuring Quality Cancer Care* (IOM, 1999), which included a recommendation to "Ensure quality of care at the end of life, in particular, the management of cancer-related and pain and timely referral to palliative and hospice care." The Board's July 2001 report *Improving Palliative Care for Cancer* further explored that mandate through a collection of commissioned papers covering economic issues, quality indicators, patient and family information, care of vulnerable populations, pediatric oncology, clinical practice guidelines, research issues and professional education. Recommendations were made in a number of those areas, but the Board deferred recommendations related to data collection until a follow-on report could evaluate (1) the capacity of currently collected data to assess care at the end of life and (2) the needs for data in the future to monitor improvement efforts. This report fills that gap.

The National Cancer Policy Board's July 2001 report on palliative care is the immediate predecessor of this report, but a broader foundation in this area had been laid by the Institute of Medicine's 1997 report *Approaching Death: Improving Care at the End of Life*. The 1997 report, produced by the Institute's Committee on Care at the End of Life, proposed a conceptual definition of a good death: one that is free from avoidable distress and suffering for patients, families, and caregivers; in general accord with patients' and families' wishes; and reasonably consistent with clinical, cultural, and ethical standards. The key components of this definition will be incorporated into the later discussion of data elements needed to monitor the quality of care at the end of life.

TABLE 1-1 Numbers of Deaths by Age
Group, 2000

All ages	2,404,598
Under 1 year	27,987
1-4 years	4,964
5-14	7,386
15-24	31,259
25-34	40,409
35-44	89,652
45-54	160,014
55-64	241,029
65-74	441,991
75-84	701,173
85 and older	658,295

SOURCE: Minino and Smith, 2001.

NUMBERS AND CAUSES OF DEATH IN THE UNITED STATES

In the year 2000, 2.4 million Americans died (Table 1-1). Most—1.8 million—were older than 65, but half a million died in early and late middle age. About 28,000 infants died before their first birthday, and 44,000 children and young adults—from age 1 to age 24—were among those who died in 2000. The patterns of mortality vary among age groups, as one would expect (Table 1-2). Heart disease and cancer predominate in older age groups, and hence, overall. Even among children and young adults, however, cancer is an important cause, and other conditions that may involve prolonged periods of decline and dying (including chronic diseases and congenital anomalies) are also significant.

Special Emphasis on Deaths of Children and Young Adults

In the United States, death in childhood is rare. This was not the case 100 years ago, and still is not in many parts of the world today, but here, death before adulthood stands out as a particular tragedy, not a commonplace event. These deaths take on far greater significance than their numbers would suggest, touching thousands more parents, siblings, grandparents, other family members, friends, neighbors, schoolmates, and professional caregivers.

In this report, we take note of how well or poorly childhood and young adult deaths are accounted for in national data collections. The numbers of these deaths are so small, they may not show up at all (or may be intentionally excluded) in sample surveys, but there is still a need and

TABLE 1-2 Top Five Causes of Death, by Age Group, 2000

Age Group Rank	Infant (<1yr)	1-4 yrs	5-14 yrs	15-24 yrs	25-44 yrs	45-64 yrs	> 65 yrs
1	Congenital anomalies (birth defects)	Accidents	Accidents	Accidents	Accidents	Cancer	Heart disease
2	Short gestation/ low birthweight	Congenital anomalies (birth defects)	Cancer	Homicide	Cancer	Heart disease	Cancer
3	Sudden infant death syndrome	Cancer	Homicide	Suicide	Heart disease	Accidents	Stroke
4	Complications of pregnancy	Homicide	Congenital anomalies	Cancer	Suicide	Stroke	Chronic lower respiratory disease
5	Respiratory distress syndrome	Heart disease	Heart disease	Heart disease	HIV infection	Pneumonia & influenza	Pneumonia & influenza

SOURCE: Minino and Smith, 2001.

a desire to understand more about the dying experiences of the young people who die and their survivors. The recommendations in Chapter 5 include ways that this can be accomplished.

OVERVIEW OF THE CURRENT REPORT

This report by the National Cancer Policy Board addresses four key questions:

1. What data would ideally inform end-of-life care?
2. What data are currently available to describe dying in America?
3. What methodological issues must be considered in the collection and use of data about dying?
4. What steps can be taken to enhance data collection efforts so that they can be used to monitor and improve the quality of end-of-life care?

To prepare this report, the Board contracted with staff at the RAND Center to Improve Care of the Dying to compile a catalog of nationally representative surveys, disease registries, administrative and billing data, and vital statistics files which could be used to describe the experience of dying in America. These datasets address the full range of ages and potential causes of death. A panel of experts critically reviewed the resulting catalog to (1) assess the extent to which existing data could be used to describe care at the end of life; (2) identify the limitations of current data collection efforts; and (3) develop strategies to improve the data available to monitor the quality of end-of-life care.

Organization of the Report

Chapter 2 describes proposed domains of quality of life and quality of care at the end of life and identifies data elements that might be available in current datasets to permit monitoring care.

Chapter 3 summarizes administrative information about the large publicly available datasets that track decedents and describes the data elements that capture information relevant to end-of-life care.

Chapter 4 outlines methodological issues, such as the generalizability of existing samples, limitations of survey methods, use of proxy data, confidentiality and linking datasets, and other issues uniquely associated with collecting information about the end of life.

Chapter 5 summarizes the report findings and presents the National Cancer Policy Board's recommendations.

2

Key Data Elements
Pertaining to the End of Life

The effort to better understand and to improve the care received by those at the end of life will require better information about dying—not just about the demographic characteristics and health conditions of those who die, but also about their quality of life as they cope with declining health, the quality of their death, and the quality of the health care provided to them during this time.

If we aim to achieve good quality of life even with declining health, and death without unnecessary suffering, undue financial burden on the family, and with respect for individual and family preferences, one of the things we must do is monitor data that provide information about these aspects of dying. Nationally representative surveys, disease registries, health care billing data and vital statistics are among the possible sources of this information. To date, most analyses of data from identified decedents has focused on factors contributing to death, rather than on the experience of dying. Thus, for example, the National Mortality Followback Surveys (NMFS) were conducted primarily to obtain information on important characteristics of the decedent that may have affected mortality (Seeman et al., 1989). The public health goal was to learn how to better prevent premature death, with the implicit assumption that almost any death could be delayed. This is evident even in the topics of the most recent (1993) NMFS, which included socioeconomic differentials in mortality and the associations between risk factors and cause of death.

To better understand dying, rather than how to delay death, a very different set of topics would be of interest, perhaps including characteristics of the site of death, symptoms and quality of life in the last year of life for patients and their families, patient preferences for and continuity of care in the last year of life, and family burden (physical, psychological, practical, and financial). The purpose of this chapter is to review the existing literature on quality of life at the end of life and quality of care at the end of life in order to identify data elements that would provide useful information about dying in America.

DEFINITION OF "THE END OF LIFE"

Designating a period of time as "the end of life" is a difficult but necessary first step. The conceptual model of a "terminal illness" has driven most current public policy about dying, though dying is not so easily predictable for most Americans. Death more frequently occurs during an exacerbation of an otherwise chronic illness or from a complication associated with a very long slow decline in old age (Lunney et al., 2001).

Although any operational definition of end of life would have to depend upon the dataset used, for the purposes of this report, the end of life is defined very broadly. In this report, the term includes the period of time during which an individual copes with declining health from an ultimately terminal illness—from a serious though perhaps chronic illness or from the frailties associated with advanced age even if death is not clearly imminent. We note that life's ending can come at any age and time, and that death at a young age is a special sorrow (IOM, 1997). Finally, we note that the terms "family" and "loved ones" will be used interchangeably in this report to connote those who have a close connection to the dying person, regardless of their genetic or legal ties.

CATEGORIES OF DATA RELEVANT TO THE QUALITY OF LIFE AND CARE OF PEOPLE AT THE END OF LIFE

Numerous public discussions and focus group research have helped us to understand what the American public values in the care of the dying (Steinhauser et al., 2000a, b; Teno et al., 2001). Domains relevant to the quality of health care and quality of life include the following:

- The management of symptoms;
- Spiritual and personal growth;
- A familiar setting, surrounded by loved ones;
- Understandable information to guide decision making and planning;
- Confidence that one will not be a financial, emotional, or physical

burden to family members; and
  • Right of self-determination, control of treatment choices.

Likewise, professional organizations have begun to identify desirable care outcomes and guidelines for practice. The National Hospice and Palliative Care Organization (NHPCO) produced a document outlining key outcomes to be targeted by hospice and palliative care groups within three domains: self-determined life closure, safe and comfortable dying, and effective grieving. Table 2-1 summarizes these outcomes. The emphasis here is close to the time of death, without emphasis on prior advance care planning and coping with declining health. Yet the specific outcomes recommended by the NHPCO also fit within the broader domains described by other authors.

In a recent paper describing the capacities and limitations of information systems as data sources on quality of care at the end of life, Nerenz proposes the following "dimensions of quality" or types of quality mea-

TABLE 2-1 National Hospice and Palliative Care Organization Recommended Outcomes

Self-determined life closure
  • Staff will prevent problems associated with coping, grieving, and existential results related to imminence of death
  • Staff will support the patient in achieving the optimal level of consciousness
  • Staff will promote adaptive behaviors that are personally effective for the patient and family caregiver

Safe and comfortable dying
  • Staff appropriately treat and prevent extension of disease and/or comorbidity
  • Staff treat and prevent treatment side effects
  • Staff treat and prevent distressing symptoms in concert with patient's wishes
  • Staff tailor treatments to patient's and family's functional capacity
  • Staff prevent crises from arising due to resource deficits
  • Staff respond appropriately to financial, legal, and environment problems that compromise care

Effective grieving
  • Staff treat and prevent coping problems
  • Staff coach the patient and family through normal grieving
  • Staff assess and respond to anticipatory grief
  • Staff prevent unnecessary premature death
  • Staff identify opportunities for family members' grief work
  • Staff assess the potential for complicated grief and respond appropriately
  • Staff assist the family in integrating the memory of their loved one into their lives

sures that would have a place in a comprehensive quality measurement system: evidence-based guidelines, adverse events (including deaths), length of survival, quality of survival, respect for preferences, and satisfaction (Nerenz, 2001).

Some investigators have modeled factors affecting the quality of care at the end of life in terms of the generally accepted framework for an assessment of quality of care—i.e., in terms of context, structure, process, and outcomes (IOM, 1997; Stewart et al., 1999). Table 2-2 provides an overview of two such models: the Institute of Medicine's model and the Stewart model.

Others in end-of-life care have focused on the identification of key domains for measurement in order to monitor quality of life and quality of care at the end of life. Emanuel has identified six "malleable inputs" or areas open to intervention by the health care system: physical symptoms, psychological symptoms, social relationships, economic and care giving responsibilities, hopes and expectations, and philosophical or spiritual beliefs (Emanuel and Emanuel, 1998). These ideas provide the basis upon which to compare domains from other sources. Teno has identified five key domains for measurement: symptom management, shared decision-making, patient satisfaction, coordination of care, and continuity of care (Teno et al., 2000; Teno, 2001). In addition to these domains, she notes the importance of family information, education, support, and bereavement support. The American Geriatrics Society adopted a list of 10 principles designed to stimulate further efforts to develop performance standards that can lead to improved care at the end of life (Lynn, 1997).

Table 2-3 presents a comparison of three such efforts—Emanuel, Teno, and the American Geriatrics Society—and forms the foundation for a selection of data categories representing information that might be found in currently existing large datasets.

The data categories identified in Table 2-3 represent information that can be expected to exist now within large data collection efforts. These elements only begin to answer the pressing questions about the end of life, including those shown in Box 2-1.

The data categories identified in Table 2-3 above and the questions posed in Box 2-1 provide a framework for the evaluation of information currently available in large datasets in Chapter 3.

TABLE 2-2 Existing Conceptual Models for Assessing Quality of Care at the End of Life

Context	Structure	Process	Outcome
IOM Model			
Culture, norms, social institutions	Care settings	Establishing diagnosis and prognosis	Physical (symptoms and function)
	Personnel		
Demographic			
	Clinical policies, protocols, guidelines	Establishing goals and plans	Psychological (emotional, cognitive)
Geography			
Economic system resources		Providing palliative and other patient care	Spiritual
	Information and decision support systems		
Political system, policies, regulations			Perception of care
		Caring for families, bereavement care	
	Financial policies		
Individual and family characteristics			Burden of care
		Coordinating care including transfers among settings	Dignity, control over decision-making
		Monitoring, improving care	Survival
Stewart Model			
Patient and family situation	Access to care within system	Technical process with patient	Patient satisfaction with care
Clinical status, case-mix	Organization of care	Decision-making process with patient and family	Family satisfaction with care
Social support for patient	Formal support services available	Information, counseling of patient and family	Quality of life of patient
Social support for family	Physical environment(s) of care		Quality of life of family and loved ones
		Interpersonal and communication style with family	Quality of dying of patient
			Length of life

TABLE 2-3 Proposed Domains and Selected Data Categories

Emanuel	Teno	American Geriatrics Society	Data Categories
Physical symptoms	Symptom management	Physical and emotional symptoms	Cause of death Comorbid conditions Physical symptoms Physical function
Psychological symptoms		Global quality of life	Psychological symptoms Quality of life Cognitive status
Social relationships		Support of function and autonomy	Household composition Site of death Social supports
Economic and caregiving responsibilities	(family information, education, support, and bereavement support)	Family burden	Family care giving Out of pocket costs Bereavement support
Hopes and expectations	Shared decision making	Advance care planning	Advance directives Decision-making
	Patient satisfaction	Patient and family expectations	Satisfaction with care Communication
		Lack of aggressive care near death	
		Survival time	
Philosophical or spiritual beliefs			Supportive services
	Coordination of care	Provider continuity and skill	Health care utilization Quality of care Quantity of care Cost of care Access to care
	Continuity of care		Provider information Service integration

---

BOX 2-1

**Questions to Assess and Monitor How Well Individuals'
End-of-Life Needs Are Being Met**

- Where are people dying and how much of the end of their lives is spent in those settings?
- Who is providing care for them as they die? Do institutional settings support family presence at the end of life?
- Are physical and psychological symptoms being identified and treated (including but not limited to pain)?
- How many persons experience impaired cognitive function before death, to what degree, and for what period of time?
- How many persons experience physical disability or social isolation before death, to what degree, and for what period of time?
- How do patients and loved ones perceive their quality of life at various time points prior to death?
- Are patients and loved ones achieving a sense of life closure?
- Are patients and loved ones involved in decision making about treatment and care options?
- Do dying persons have adequate access to supportive end-of-life care?
- What forms of health care delivery are most helpful in promoting end-of-life care goals?
- Are patients and loved ones able to make informed decisions based on timely and adequate information about what to expect, treatment options, services, and resources?
- Are patients and loved ones receiving supportive services from chaplains, therapists, health aides, and other providers?
- Are family physical, emotional, and financial resources being heavily depleted by the care of a dying family member? Are burdens spread across many or borne by a few?
- Are loved ones supported through the grieving process?

3

Currently Available Datasets

This chapter describes ongoing surveys and other data collection efforts that include information about decedents. It describes (1) datasets traditionally used to describe dying; (2) Census Bureau surveys; (3) national health surveys; (4) surveys focused on the elderly; (5) disease registries and surveillance studies; (6) reimbursement-specific administrative databases; and (7) other data collected by and about health care organizations. This chapter describes the original purpose of each data source and a brief overview of the way in which the information gathered could contribute to an improved understanding of dying in America. The appendices provide details about the sample, information about the timeframe of data collection, and availability of the data, questionnaires and coding instructions for these data sources, as well as a bibliography of publications derived from the data. The chapter concludes with a discussion of the information most readily available from existing datasets and the limitations of these data in answering the important questions about the end of life that were posed at the end of Chapter 2.

There are a number of ways to arrange the data sources described in this chapter. They are ordered with those most relevant to death and dying first, and the more general surveys, with some information of interest, later. All the entries are also listed in Table 3-1, which has a code for the nature of each data set—e.g., administrative, national health survey—in addition to noting the numbers of deaths covered and the types of information collected.

DATASETS TRADITIONALLY USED TO DESCRIBE DYING

Death Certificates

The most immediate information gathered about a death is found on the state-required death certificate. National vital statistics rely heavily on information from death certificates, although federal tracking of death registration was not complete across the entire United States until 1933 (Lilienfeld and Lilienfield, 1980). The U.S. Standard Certificate of Death (Figure 3-1) was developed through a collaborative effort between the National Center for Health Statistics and the states. Although there is no formal agreement to use this standard certificate, the National Center for Health Statistics has an agreement with the states through the Vital Statistics Cooperative Program to provide data in specified formats consistent with the standard certificate.

The death certificate assigns physicians, medical examiners, and coroners the responsibility for documenting the cause of death through a system that acknowledges the possibility of multiple causes. The disease, injury or complication that caused death (not the mode of dying such as a cardiac arrest) is noted on line "a" as the immediate cause of death. Then diseases or injuries that initiated the events resulting in death are recorded, beginning with the condition that gave rise to the immediate cause of death (line b), which in turn resulted from a further condition (line c). Additional lines may be added as necessary such that the underlying cause of death is on the lowest line used in Part I. Part II of the death certificate is used to list other significant conditions contributing to death but not resulting in the underlying cause of death. Demographic data (such as age, race, place of residence and marital status) and crude measures of socioeconomic status (SES) (such as educational attainment, usual occupation, kind of business) are recorded by the funeral director on the death certificate.

The National Center for Health Statistics will recommend a revised version of the standard death certificate in 2003, which will include the expansion of the question on Place of Death to include "Hospice Facility." Although problems with improper completion of death certificates and inaccuracy in reporting the cause of death continue (Lloyd-Jones et al., 1998; Maudsley and Williams, 1996; Smith Sehdev and Hutchins, 2001), the National Center for Health Statistics continues to develop and advance standardized coding, training workshops and other quality improvement efforts. Part of the problem is the lack of formal training in many medical schools or residency programs. Further, there is considerable variation among states in the sophistication of record keeping, in-

TABLE 3-1 Types of Data Available from Datasets That Contain Individual-Level Information

Data type		Number of deaths year[s]	Cause of death	Comorbidities	Pain or other physical symptoms
C2	AHEAD	1,900 (1993-98)		✓	✓
C2	LSOA I & II	I: 2,900 (1984-90) II: 1,900 (1994-2000)	✓	✓	
C1	MCBS	700/yr		✓	
B	MDS			✓	✓
B	Medicare claims	1.7 million (2000)		✓	
C1	MEPS	NA²		✓	✓
A	Death Certificates (NDI)	2.4 M (2000)	✓		
C1	NHANES	50/yr estimate		✓	✓
C2	NHEFS	1,400 (1987-92)¹	✓	✓	✓
C2	NHHCS	~5,000 (2000)		✓	
C1	NHIS	55,000 (1986-94)		✓	✓
C2	NLTCS	17,000 (1982-86)		✓	
C2	NMFS	23,000 (1993)	✓	✓	
C1	NNHS	~1,600 (1999)		✓	
B	OASIS			✓	✓
C1	PSID	4,300 (thru 1999)		✓	

Physical function	Psychological symptoms	QoL	Cognition	Site of death	Lived with	Social support
✓	✓	✓	✓		✓	✓
✓				✓	✓	✓
✓			✓		✓	✓
✓	✓		✓		✓	✓
✓	✓		✓		✓	
				✓		
✓			✓		✓	
✓				✓	✓	
✓					✓	
✓	✓		✓		✓	
✓	✓		✓		✓	✓
✓			✓	✓	✓	
✓					✓	
✓	✓		✓		✓	
✓					✓	

TABLE 3-1 Continued

Data type		Family care	Out of pocket expenses	Bereavement	ADS
C2	AHEAD	✓	✓		✓
C2	LSOA I & II	✓			✓
C1	MCBS		✓		
B	MDS		✓		✓
B	Medicare claims				
C1	MEPS	✓	✓		
A	Death Certificates (NDI)				
C1	NHANES				
C2	NHEFS				
C2	NHHCS	✓	✓		
C1	NHIS		✓		
C2	NLTCS	✓	✓		✓
C2	NMFS	✓	✓		✓
C1	NNHS		✓		
B	OASIS	✓			
C1	PSID	✓			

KEY: First Column: A = Vital statistics; B = Administrative data; C = Research sample (C1 = continuous or regular sample; C2 = not continuous or regularly occurring sample); AHEAD—Asset and Health Dynamics Among the Oldest Old; LSOA—Longitudinal Survey of Aging; MCBS—Medicare Current Beneficiary Survey; MDS—nursing home Minimum Data Set; MEPS—Medicare Expenditure Panel Survey; NDI—National Death Index; NHANES—National Health and Nutrition Examination Survey; NHEFS—NHANES I Epidemiologic Followup Survey; NHHCS—National Home and Hospice Care Survey; NHIS—National Health Interview Survey; NLTCS—National

cluding the use of electronic records. The use of death certificate information will be greatly facilitated as the National Center for Health Statistics works in collaboration with the states to build a totally electronic infrastructure to collect and manage these data.

Decision making	Satisfaction	Support	Use of services	Quality	Provider
			✓		
			✓		
	✓	✓	✓	✓	
		✓	✓		
			✓		✓
	✓	✓	✓	✓	✓
			✓		
			✓		
		✓	✓		
			✓	✓	
		✓	✓		
✓		✓	✓	✓	
		✓			✓
		✓	✓		✓
			✓		

Long-Term Care Survey; NMFS—National Mortality Followback Survey; NNHS—National Nursing Home Survey; OASIS—Outcome and Assessment Information Set; PSID—Panel Study of Income Dynamics.

[1]Deaths during 5-year follow-up period total 20-year follow-up (1971-1992).
[2]MEPS data will be linked to the NDI when a large enough number of deaths have occurred. It is currently too early for this.

National Death Index (NDI)

The NDI is a central computerized index of death certificate information that was established as a resource for epidemiologists and other health researchers to determine if persons in their studies have died. The NDI provides researchers with the state where death occurred and the

TYPE/PRINT IN PERMANENT BLACK INK		U.S. STANDARD **CERTIFICATE OF DEATH**				
FOR INSTRUCTIONS SEE OTHER SIDE AND HANDBOOK	LOCAL FILE NUMBER			STATE FILE NUMBER		

Items below reproduced as a structured form:

DECEDENT

- 1. DECEDENT'S NAME *(First, Middle, Last)* | 2. SEX | 3. DATE OF DEATH *(Month, Day, Year)*
- 4. SOCIAL SECURITY NUMBER | 5a. AGE—Last Birthday *(Years)* | 5b. UNDER 1 YEAR — Months / Days | 5c. UNDER 1 DAY — Hours / Minutes | 6. DATE OF BIRTH *(Month, Day, Year)* | 7. BIRTHPLACE *(City and State or Foreign Country)*
- 8. WAS DECEDENT EVER IN U.S. ARMED FORCES? *(Yes or no)* | 9a. PLACE OF DEATH *(Check only one; see instructions on other side)* HOSPITAL: □ Inpatient □ ER/Outpatient □ DOA OTHER: □ Nursing Home □ Residence □ Other *(Specify)*
- 9b. FACILITY NAME *(If not institution, give street and number)* | 9c. CITY, TOWN, OR LOCATION OF DEATH | 9d. COUNTY OF DEATH
- 10. MARITAL STATUS—Married, Never Married, Widowed, Divorced *(Specify)* | 11. SURVIVING SPOUSE *(If wife, give maiden name)* | 12a. DECEDENT'S USUAL OCCUPATION *(Give kind of work done during most of working life. Do not use retired.)* | 12b. KIND OF BUSINESS/INDUSTRY
- 13a. RESIDENCE—STATE | 13b. COUNTY | 13c. CITY, TOWN, OR LOCATION | 13d. STREET AND NUMBER
- 13e. INSIDE CITY LIMITS? *(Yes or no)* | 13f. ZIP CODE | 14. WAS DECEDENT OF HISPANIC ORIGIN? *(Specify No or Yes—If yes, specify Cuban, Mexican, Puerto Rican, etc.)* □ No □ Yes Specify: | 15. RACE—American Indian, Black, White, etc. *(Specify)* | 16. DECEDENT'S EDUCATION *(Specify only highest grade completed)* Elementary/Secondary (0-12) | College (1-4 or 5+)

PARENTS

- 17. FATHER'S NAME *(First, Middle, Last)* | 18. MOTHER'S NAME *(First, Middle, Maiden Surname)*

INFORMANT

- 19a. INFORMANT'S NAME *(Type/Print)* | 19b. MAILING ADDRESS *(Street and Number or Rural Route Number, City or Town, State, Zip Code)*

DISPOSITION

- 20a. METHOD OF DISPOSITION □ Burial □ Cremation □ Removal from State □ Donation □ Other *(Specify)* | 20b. PLACE OF DISPOSITION *(Name of cemetery, crematory, or other place)* | 20c. LOCATION—City or Town, State
- 21a. SIGNATURE OF FUNERAL SERVICE LICENSEE OR PERSON ACTING AS SUCH ▶ | 21b. LICENSE NUMBER *(of Licensee)* | 22. NAME AND ADDRESS OF FACILITY

PRONOUNCING PHYSICIAN ONLY — ITEMS 24-26 MUST BE COMPLETED BY PERSON WHO PRONOUNCES DEATH

- Complete items 23a-c only when certifying physician is not available at time of death to certify cause of death. | 23a. To the best of my knowledge, death occurred at the time, date, and place stated. Signature and Title ▶ | 23b. LICENSE NUMBER | 23c. DATE SIGNED *(Month, Day, Year)*
- 24. TIME OF DEATH ___ M | 25. DATE PRONOUNCED DEAD *(Month, Day, Year)* | 26. WAS CASE REFERRED TO MEDICAL EXAMINER/CORONER? *(Yes or no)*

CAUSE OF DEATH

- 27. PART I. Enter the diseases, injuries, or complications that caused the death. Do not enter the mode of dying, such as cardiac or respiratory arrest, shock, or heart failure. List only one cause on each line. | Approximate Interval Between Onset and Death
  - IMMEDIATE CAUSE (Final disease or condition resulting in death) ▶ a. _____ DUE TO (OR AS A CONSEQUENCE OF):
  - Sequentially list conditions, if any, leading to immediate cause. Enter UNDERLYING CAUSE (Disease or injury that initiated events resulting in death) LAST ▶ b. _____ DUE TO (OR AS A CONSEQUENCE OF): c. _____ DUE TO (OR AS A CONSEQUENCE OF): d. _____
- PART II. Other significant conditions contributing to death but not resulting in the underlying cause given in Part I. | 28a. WAS AN AUTOPSY PERFORMED? *(Yes or no)* | 28b. WERE AUTOPSY FINDINGS AVAILABLE PRIOR TO COMPLETION OF CAUSE OF DEATH? *(Yes or no)*
- 29. MANNER OF DEATH □ Natural □ Accident □ Suicide □ Homicide □ Pending Investigation □ Could not be Determined | 30a. DATE OF INJURY *(Month, Day, Year)* | 30b. TIME OF INJURY ___ M | 30c. INJURY AT WORK? *(Yes or no)* | 30d. DESCRIBE HOW INJURY OCCURRED
- 30e. PLACE OF INJURY—At home, farm, street, factory, office building, etc. *(Specify)* | 30f. LOCATION *(Street and Number or Rural Route Number, City or Town, State)*

CERTIFIER

- 31a. CERTIFIER *(Check only one)*
  - □ CERTIFYING PHYSICIAN *(Physician certifying cause of death when another physician has pronounced death and completed Item 23)* To the best of my knowledge, death occurred due to the cause(s) and manner as stated.
  - □ PRONOUNCING AND CERTIFYING PHYSICIAN *(Physician both pronouncing death and certifying to cause of death)* To the best of my knowledge, death occurred at the time, date, and place, and due to the cause(s) and manner as stated.
  - □ MEDICAL EXAMINER/CORONER On the basis of examination and/or investigation, in my opinion, death occurred at the time, date, and place, and due to the cause(s) and manner as stated.
- 31b. SIGNATURE AND TITLE OF CERTIFIER ▶ | 31c. LICENSE NUMBER | 31d. DATE SIGNED *(Month, Day, Year)*
- 32. NAME AND ADDRESS OF PERSON WHO COMPLETED CAUSE OF DEATH (ITEM 27) *(Type/Print)*

REGISTRAR

- 33. REGISTRAR'S SIGNATURE | 34. DATE FILED *(Month, Day, Year)*

PHS-T-003

Left margin: NAME OF DECEDENT: For use by physician or institution — SEE INSTRUCTIONS ON OTHER SIDE — SEE DEFINITION ON OTHER SIDE — SEE INSTRUCTIONS ON OTHER SIDE — SEE DEFINITION ON OTHER SIDE — DEPARTMENT OF HEALTH AND HUMAN SERVICES – PUBLIC HEALTH SERVICE – NATIONAL CENTER FOR HEALTH STATISTICS – 1989 REVISION

FIGURE 3-1 Standard U.S. Death Certificate.

death certificate number, which researchers use to obtain death certificate information directly from the appropriate state. To use the system, investigators must first submit an application to the National Center for Health Statistics. Fees are based on a service charge plus a fee for each user record for each year of death searched.

National Mortality Followback Surveys (NMFS)

The NMFS supplement information on death certificates with information on important characteristics of decedents. Information is collected from proxy next-of-kin informants identified on the death certificate. First instituted in the early 1960s, the various NMFS have been collaborative projects between the National Center for Health Statistics and various federal, state, and local organizations. To date, there have been six surveys (1961, 1962-1963, 1964-1965, 1966-1968, 1986, 1993) designed to provide information about the use of health services prior to death, socioeconomic status, aspects of life style, and other factors that may affect when and how death occurs. The 1986 NMFS file consisted of four types of linked records for 18,733 decedents, including (1) data from death certificates; (2) proxy surveys; (3) the medical examiners file for deaths due to homicide, suicide, and accidents; and (4) information from health care facilities used in the last year of life. The 1993 NMFS was based on a sample of 22,957 death certificates and focused on socioeconomic differentials in mortality and the prevention of premature death. The 1993 NMFS excluded deaths of people under age 15. For this survey, additional information was collected about risk factors and disability. No future surveys are currently being planned.

National Longitudinal Mortality Study (NLMS)

The NLMS is a large study of the effects of occupation, industry, income, education, and other socioeconomic factors on mortality. Records from several Current Population Surveys of the Bureau of the Census (1979-1981) have been matched to the National Death Index to link individual social and economic data with mortality outcomes. While the focus of this is on mortality, rather than quality or care of dying, the published reports do enhance our understanding of the role of social and economic variables on the age at death (Backlund et al., 1999; Johnson et al., 2000; Kaufman and Kaufman, 2001). This effort also highlights the value of linking the National Death Index with large ongoing national data collection efforts. The Current Population Surveys include only individuals age 16 and older, so no children are represented in the dataset linked to the National Death Index.

Medicare Data

Medicare Claims Data

Medicare claims data also contribute to our understanding of dying. More than 80 percent of American decedents received health care under Medicare, either because they qualified by being at least 65 years old or because they were disabled or had end-stage renal disease (Hogan et al., 2001). In addition to the various Medicare claims files, the Medicare Continuous History File contains Medicare beneficiaries' basic entitlement data as well as Part A and Part B detailed claims (which include CPT and procedure codes). It is available continuously for 5 percent of all Medicare beneficiaries, or more than 1.5 million individuals in any given year. The entitlement file is linked to decedent records derived from the Social Security Administration. Approximately 5 percent of Medicare beneficiaries die in any given year. While the range of beneficiary characteristics is limited to age, sex, race, and geographical region, a wide array of health care utilization variables can be derived from the records of hospitalizations; stays in skilled nursing facilities; hospice services; and outpatient clinic, physician, and home health visits. These data have been used extensively to describe the intensity of medical services in the year preceding death (Virnig et al., 1999a,b, 2000, 2001, 2002; Christakis and Escarce, 1996; Christakis and Iwashyna, 2000). However, it should be noted that there are important gaps because of the lack of specific data about care delivered to beneficiaries receiving capitated HMO or hospice services. The only administrative data available in those cases is the amount paid per contract (in the case of the HMO) or per day (for hospice). Approximately 20 percent of deaths among Medicare beneficiaries occur under the hospice benefit. The current lack of detail about the specific services or medications received during that care within Medicare claims data hampers the ability to evaluate the quality of that care. Minor increases in the data elements on these claims forms would provide a means to evaluate the content of care and begin to assess quality.

A small number of children are eligible for Medicare because of disability, but this would be a negligible source of information about children who die. However, Medicaid data are available about deaths among children covered by that program (discussed later in this chapter).

Medicare Current Beneficiary Survey (MCBS)

Within the Medicare program, the Centers for Medicare and Medicaid Services (CMS)—formerly known as the Health Care Financing Administration—conducts the MCBS, a continuous, multipurpose survey of a representative national sample of the Medicare population, including those living in institutions. The purpose of the MCBS is to determine health care expenditures and sources of payments for all services beneficiaries use (including non-Medicare covered services) and to trace changes in health status and spending over time.

Participants are interviewed in person for about an hour every four months, for up to four years (at which time they are replaced by new interviewees). At each interview, they are asked about their use of health services, medical care expenditures, health insurance coverage, and sources of payment (public and private, including out-of-pocket payments). Other questions are asked once each year, including information of relevance to this report, on health status and functioning. If the person is unable to answer the survey questions, he or she is asked to designate a proxy respondent, usually a family member or close acquaintance who is familiar with his or her care. About 15 percent of the interviews of non-institutionalized individuals are with proxy respondents. The data are designed to support both cross-sectional and longitudinal analyses and can be linked to Medicare claims data.

The first round of interviews was conducted in 1991, and the survey has been in the field continuously since then. The target sample for the MCBS is 12,000 persons with three years of cost and use information. The MCBS includes roughly 700 decedents each year (Hogan et al., 2000) and adds important information about health care utilization and functioning prior to death.

CENSUS BUREAU SURVEYS

Although the datasets described above have been the ones most traditionally used to describe dying in America, many others have the potential to add to our understanding of end-of-life issues. Data collected by the U.S. Bureau of the Census provide general statistical information about the condition of the country and its population.

Census 2000

From the decennial Census 2000, information is available on about 115.9 million housing units and 281.4 million people. Although the primary purpose of the census is to identify demographic trends, two questions about disability were included in the Census 2000 long form that provide a general picture of physical impairment within the population. In approximately one out of six households, the respondent was asked about the presence of a long-lasting condition that limited basic physical activities such as walking, climbing stairs, reaching, lifting, or carrying. A second question addressed difficulty learning, remembering, concentrating, dressing, bathing or getting around inside the home.

Other Census Bureau Surveys

The Census Bureau continually conducts surveys throughout the decade between censuses to track social and economic conditions. These include the following:

- **Current Population Survey (CPS).** The CPS is a monthly survey of 50,000 households, is primarily targeted to provide information on the labor force of individuals age 16 and older (i.e., no children). However, CPS questions also address disability, and recent supplements included a Health/Pension survey in 1994. A regular supplement deals with health insurance coverage.
- **Survey of Income and Program Participation (SIPP).** The SIPP is another source of information on disability from the Census Bureau. The SIPP is a longitudinal panel survey of non-institutionalized adults, in which approximately 14,000 households are entered at the beginning of each calendar year and interviewed at specific intervals over a 2- to 3-year period of time. An extensive set of disability questions was asked in the 1990, 1991, 1992, 1993, 1996, and 2000 panels.

Although the data from these surveys conducted by the Census Bureau have limited direct value in understanding quality of life or care at the end of life, the sampling strategies established by the Census Bureau are the foundation for most federal surveys. The coordination of federal surveys is an efficient way of ensuring that samples will be representative of the national population and that individual households will not be burdened with multiple federal surveys. The Census Bureau applies oversampling techniques to improve precision for racial and ethnic minorities and other demographically defined domains.

NATIONAL HEALTH SURVEYS

Large federal health surveys are also useful to understanding what happens at the end of life. There is likely to be substantial variation in the health of persons in the months and years before death, but surprisingly little published data support this assumption. Examining the information provided by respondents to health surveys who later die will begin to fill this gap. For example, beginning with the survey year 1986, the National Center for Health Statistics collected linkage information on all respondents to the National Health Interview Survey (NHIS), described below, to permit matching to the National Death Index. Among respondents to the surveys between 1986 and 1994, there have been 54,534 adults subsequently identified as deceased (Schoeni et al., 2002). More than 10,000 of these people died within two years of their health interview. (Children have been excluded from this linkage.)

National Health Interview Survey (NHIS)

Data from the NHIS could be analyzed to improve our understanding of health and functioning at the end of life. The NHIS, a cross-sectional survey, is the principal source of information on the health of the civilian, non-institutionalized household population of the United States. It has been conducted continuously since 1957 and data are released in public use files on an annual basis. The interviewed sample for 2000 consisted of 38,633 households, which yielded information on 100,618 persons (90 percent household response rate). In-depth interviews (the "Sample Adult component") was completed by 32,374 people 18 years and older, and proxy interviews (with someone age 18 or older) were completed for 13,376 children under age 18. The general health measures in the basic module include health behaviors, health conditions, limitations of activity, and health care access and utilization.

In the mid-1990s, the U.S. Department of Health and Human Services (HHS) began a series of activities designed to better integrate national health related data collection efforts. Prior to that point, the operation of surveys throughout the HHS was decentralized, with limited central strategic planning and direction. This resulted in a large loss of analytic benefit. In 1995, the HHS Data Council submitted a survey consolidation framework to streamline and rationalize data activities. One result was that the NHIS now serves as a sampling "nucleus" for many HHS population surveys. And the links between or among each of these surveys and the National Death Index greatly increase their utility for the purpose of better understanding how, when, and why Americans die.

National Health and Nutrition Examination Survey (NHANES)

The NHANES now uses the NHIS as its sampling frame and has links to Medicare and the National Death Index records that permit longitudinal and historical studies of disease. It provides important and detailed data to measure the prevalence and comorbidity of diseases and disorders and is unique in that it combines a home interview together with clinical data collected in a mobile examination center. The detailed data include information about medical conditions, pain, cardiovascular fitness, physical activity and functioning, social support, diet behavior and nutrition, and housing characteristics.

Unfortunately the relatively small sample size is a serious limitation for the purpose of studying decedents. Approximately 5,000 people are examined each in 12-month period, and since 1999, each annual sample is representative of the entire U.S. population (i.e., not just adults or older people). The U.S. crude death rate (877 deaths per 100,000) suggests that even data pooled over a 10-year period from this survey would yield only 500 deaths (and very few deaths among children). Nonetheless, the rich clinical detail in this survey warrants its consideration for studying some deaths among adults.

NHANES I Epidemiologic Followup Study (NHEFS)

The NHEFS was a longitudinal study that used as its baseline the 14,400 adults who were examined in the first NHANES panel (1971-1975). The objectives of the NHEFS were to study morbidity and mortality associated with suspected risk factors, changes over time in participants' characteristics, and the natural history of chronic disease and functional impairments. Almost 4500 of the original cohort had died by the time of the last follow-up, in 1992. Death certificate information is available for most of those. Of those subjects still alive to be included in second (1987) follow-up interviews, 1,392 were deceased by 1992. Death certificates were obtained for 1,374 of these decedents, and proxy interviews conducted for 1,130.

Although not an ongoing data collection, the NHEFS dataset is richly detailed with information about these 1,392 decedents. Children were excluded from this analysis, but the relatively small size of NHANES populations suggests that little information could be gained from it about childhood deaths.

Medical Expenditure Panel Survey (MEPS)

MEPS is now linked to the NHIS and is a nationally representative survey of health care use, expenditures, sources of payment, and insurance coverage for the U.S. civilian non-institutionalized population, as well as a national survey of nursing homes and their residents. MEPS is the third in a series of national probability surveys about the financing and utilization of medical care in the United States. The first National Medical Care Expenditure Survey (NMES-1 or NMCES) was conducted in 1977, and NMES-2 in 1986.

Information is collected on health status and disability directly within the MEPS, and is also available by the links to the NHIS. MEPS comprises four component surveys: the Household Component (HC), the Medical Provider Component (MPC), the Insurance Component (IC), and the Nursing Home Component (NHC). The MEPS HC collects data continuously at both the person and household levels through an overlapping panel design. Two calendar years of information are collected from each household in a series of five rounds of data collection over a two-year period.

In 1996, the first year of the redesigned survey, data were collected on approximately 10,000 families and 24,000 individuals in 195 communities (a sample drawn from the NHIS). The redesigned survey has the potential to be linked to the National Death Index, but to date this linkage has not been achieved because the accrued sample is too small to yield a large number of decedents. Since children are included in MEPS, they should eventually be included in any linkage studies, even though the numbers are likely to be quite small.

SURVEYS FOCUSED ON THE ELDERLY

Longitudinal Study of Aging (LSOA)

The LSOA is a family of surveys designed to measure changes in health status, health-related behaviors, health care, and the causes and consequences of these changes within and across two cohorts of elderly Americans.

• The **Supplement on Aging (SOA)** was conducted as part of the 1984 National Health Interview Survey (NHIS) on a probability sample of 16,148 persons 55 years of age and older living in the community. Those in this cohort who were 70 years of age and older were re-interviewed in three follow-up waves, conducted in 1986, 1988, and 1990.
• The **Second Supplement on Aging (SOAII)** was part of the 1994 NHIS and comprises 9,447 persons who had turned 70 by the time of the SOAII interview. This second cohort was re-interviewed between 1997-98 and again between 1999-2000.

LSOA data allow us to describe the continuum from functional independence in the community through dependence, including institutionalization, to death. There are approximately 2,867 decedents identified within the publicly available dataset from the LSOA I cohort (Wolinsky et al., 1995). The LSOA II sample has yet to be matched to National Death Index records, but by the final wave of interviewing, 1,900 persons were reported deceased (Weeks, 2001).

Health and Retirement Study (HRS) and Asset and Health Dynamics Among the Oldest Old (AHEAD) Study

The HRS, fielded first in 1992, focuses primarily on factors affecting retirement, health insurance, savings, and economic well-being. The target population first included household residents in the contiguous United States born during the years 1931-1941. The original HRS panel consisted of 12,600 persons in 7,600 households.

AHEAD studies examine the implications of health dynamics in old age for transitions in economic well-being, changes in family and marital status, and for reliance on public and private support systems. The target population for the first AHEAD survey, fielded in 1993, consisted of U.S. household residents who were born in 1923 or before. The original AHEAD study sample consisted of 7,447 HRS respondents aged 70+. AHEAD data provide information on the costs of illness borne by the family and the effectiveness of varying care arrangements in preserving function and delaying institutionalization.

In 1998, the HRS and AHEAD studies were combined to provide a rich longitudinal dataset concerned with the health, economics, and demography of aging. For the combined study, a sample of "War Babies" (born between 1942 and 1947) and a sample of "Children of the Depression" (born between 1924 and 1930) have been added. Respondents are followed longitudinally at 2-year intervals until they die. At the time of the 1998 interviews, about 1,900 of the original AHEAD participants had died.

National Long-Term Care Surveys (NLTCS)

The NLTCS are surveys of the entire aged population with a particular emphasis on the aged who are functionally impaired. The samples are drawn from Medicare beneficiary enrollment files and are nationally representative of both community and institutionalized residents. A screening questionnaire identifies elders with functional disabilities and those so identified are followed until death. Medicare records are continuously added to each person's data file through an automatic linking process.

To date, four surveys make up this collection: 1982, 1984, 1989, and 1994. Each contains a longitudinal follow-up of previously surveyed disabled elders as well as screening for additional Medicare recipients with disabilities. A supplemental survey of caregivers was fielded in 1989 and 1999, though comparisons over time are difficult because of changes in the survey. Approximately 17,000 deaths have been identified from Medicare administrative records for respondents interviewed between 1982 and 1996. A next-of-kin supplemental survey was conducted as part of the 1994 NLTCS, for the estimated 4,800 persons who died between 1989 and 1994.

Panel Study of Income Dynamics (PSID)

The PSID is a recurring national survey focused on economic and demographic issues. The major source of funding is the National Science Foundation, with additional sponsorship by NIH and other government agencies. The survey is conducted from the Survey Research Center, Institute for Social Research, University of Michigan. A wide variety of information is collected at the family and individual level about family composition, childbirth, and residential location. Over the life of the survey, the National Institute on Aging has funded supplements on health, wealth, parental health and long term care, and the financial impact of illness. For example, in 1993 the PSID interview included detailed information concerning the health events of the elderly and their burden on immediate and extended families. As a general rule, prior to 1999 only global health questions had been asked; for 1999 and 2001, much greater detail on specific health conditions is included in the health module. The PSID has gathered data about the fact and date of death of many former PSID respondents during 1993 and 1994 efforts to recontact former respondents, and through use of the NDI.

During the 1990 interviewing wave, in conjunction with an NIA-funded project, respondents age 55 or older who indicated they were Medicare beneficiaries were asked to sign permission forms for access to their 1984-1990 Medicare claim records. Those who agreed were asked to renew that permission verbally in 1991 and in following years for later Medicare claims. About 4,300 deaths had been recorded through 1999, and updates through 2001 will be made soon. The questionnaire information on out-of-pocket medical expenditures and the long time-series of core PSID information are being linked to Medicare claims data, and should result in a valuable data set.

DISEASE REGISTRIES AND SURVEILLANCE STUDIES

Disease registries provide targeted information about those with specific health conditions. Examples of these are the Surveillance, Epidemiology, and End Results (SEER) Program of the National Cancer Institute and the Framingham Heart Studies.

Surveillance, Epidemiology, and End Results (SEER) Program

The National Cancer Institute's SEER Program has been collecting and publishing cancer incidence and survival data from 11 population-based cancer registries and three supplemental registries which together cover approximately 14 percent of the U.S. population. In 2001, the program expanded, adding several registries and expanding existing ones, which increased coverage to one-quarter of the U.S. population.

The database currently contains information on more than 3 million cancer cases, and approximately 170,000 new cases are added each year. There were 5,689 cases recorded among children and young adults age 19 and under during the 5-year period 1993 through 1997, or roughly 1,000 cases per year (NCI, 2002). SEER registries routinely collect data about patient demographics, primary tumor site, morphology, stage at diagnosis, first course of treatment, and vital status follow-up. By itself, SEER registry data do not provide information on the overall quality of care or quality of life of individuals, but because it is population based, it does provide a solid sampling frame for further investigations, particularly when linked to other data sets. SEER data have been linked to the National Death Index and Medicare claims data, but the potential for other linkages exists.

REIMBURSEMENT-SPECIFIC ADMINISTRATIVE DATABASES

Although the use of data from the Medicare program was described earlier, there are other major sources of administrative data linked to reimbursement systems. All the systems are large, but none is representative of the population as a whole (as the Medicare system is for people over 65):

• **State-specific Medicaid claims data** are available from states and the Centers for Medicare and Medicaid Services (CMS) (formerly known as the Health Care Financing Administration). Although detail may be missing for some persons enrolled in managed care, the remaining data elements are detailed and quite accurate (Arnett, 1998). Unlike Medicare, however, longitudinal tracking of individuals is unreliable, because people often enroll and disenroll in Medicaid, and may move from state to state.

• **Administrative data from private insurers** are available. Large private insurers such as Blue Cross/Blue Shield and UnitedHealth Group maintain comprehensive claims databases, as do commercial vendors such as MEDSTAT/SysteMetrics, Inc. and Shared Medical Systems, Inc. (Arnett, 1998; Paul et al., 1993). Data from private insurers, because they are generally employer based, would be the best sources of information about health care for children, young and middle-aged adults who die. Data from private insurers vary in the level of detail regarding information on cost, diagnoses and procedures, and enrollment.

• **Administrative data from the Defense Department and the De-**

partment of Veterans Affairs include the following (these include virtually no children and very few women in the VA system):

—The *Defense Medical Information System (DMIS)* contains patient data with data elements comparable to those found on the National Hospital Discharge Survey (reported in the next section).

—Health-related data files maintained by the Veterans Health Administration include the *Patient Treatment File (PTF)*—patient-specific claims type data for care received at VA facilities, including admission date, diagnosis, and procedures; the *Outpatient Care File*; and the *Long-Term Care Patient Assessment Instrument File.* The VA system tracks drug prescriptions in a centralized system, so it can be very helpful in studying the use of drugs by people with particular conditions (or, e.g., in the period before death).

OTHER DATA COLLECTED BY AND ABOUT HEALTH CARE ORGANIZATIONS

Data collected on a national level by health care organizations are another potentially important source of information about dying. Health care agencies collect these data to both understand the characteristics of the clients served and to monitor the quality of care provided. Such data allow us to use aggregated characteristics of those who are cared for and who die in various types of health care agencies to better understand patterns of end-of-life care.

National Health Care Survey (NHCS)

The National Center for Health Statistics merged and expanded its surveys of health care centers into one integrated survey of health care providers called the NHCS. The NHCS builds upon and now includes the National Hospital Discharge Survey, the National Ambulatory Medical Care Survey, the National Nursing Home Survey, and the National Health Provider Inventory.

National Home and Hospice Care Survey (NHHCS)

The new package also includes the NHHCS, which is of particular relevance to this report. The NHHCS is a continuing series of surveys of home and hospice care agencies in the United States. Data are collected through personal interviews with administrators and staff and include information that profiles the clients served at the time of the survey. Client data include referral and length of service, diagnoses, number of visits, patient charges, health status, reason for discharge, and types of services provided. The 1998 NHHCS sample consisted of 1,088 agencies.

National Hospital Discharge Survey (NHDS)

The NHDS, conducted annually since 1965, collects data from a sample of approximately 270,000 inpatient records acquired from a national sample of about 500 hospitals. Data about patients include demographic information, length of stay, and medical information about diagnoses and procedures. In 1996, deaths accounted for 3 percent of all discharges (which would include only a few children). Every state has hospital discharge datasets and these are useful in examining deaths occurring within hospitals.

Healthcare Cost and Utilization Project (HCUP)

The HCUP is a federal-state-industry partnership created to build a standardized, multi-state health data system. It comprises a family of administrative longitudinal databases that contain patient-level information in a uniform format with privacy protections in place:

- The **Nationwide Inpatient Sample (NIS)** includes inpatient data from a national sample of over 1,000 hospitals.
- The **State Inpatient Databases (SID)** cover inpatient care in community hospitals in 22 states that represent more than half of all U.S. hospital discharges.
- The **State Ambulatory Surgery Databases (SASD)**, the project's newest phase, currently provides data from ambulatory care encounters in nine states. Variables include primary and secondary diagnoses and procedures, admission and discharge status, demographics, charges, and length of stay.

The uniform data in the HCUP are designed to facilitate comparative studies of health care services and the use and cost of these services. The HCUP also has been a powerful resource for the development of tools such as the Clinical Classifications Software, Comorbidity Software and the HCUP Quality Indicators. Children are included in these databases, but they would probably yield relatively little about children who die.

Nursing Home Minimum Data Set (MDS)

The nursing home MDS resident assessment and care screening system has evolved from a long-standing recognition that comprehensive functional assessment of nursing home residents is central to maximizing their physical functioning and quality of life. The development of a uniform, comprehensive resident assessment system was one of the key recommendations of the 1986 report of the Institute of Medicine's Committee on Nursing Home Regulation.

In 1990, the Health Care Financing Administration (now known as the Centers for Medicare and Medicaid Services, or CMS) published a *Resident Assessment Instrument (RAI)* and specified that assessments would be conducted on each Medicaid certified nursing home resident upon admission, upon "significant change" in status, and at least annually after admission or significant change. Beginning in 1998, all nursing home facilities were required to automate and transmit MDS information to the states, which were required to forward it to the Health Care Financing Administration (HCFA, 1998).

The MDS potentially offers a very rich resource of clinical information regarding nursing home residents' functional status, health conditions, services received, demographic characteristics, and other items such as the presence of advanced directives and family participation. As reliability trials have demonstrated, however, nursing facility staff can produce research-quality data, but, in practice, facilities differ in their commitment to ensuring that staff are trained and that they adhere to assessment protocols (Hawes et al., 1995). Furthermore, in spite of the mandate to perform an assessment with each change in status, there is wide variation in the timing of assessments prior to the death of a nursing home resident.

Outcome and Assessment Information Set (OASIS)

OASIS was developed for the purposes of measuring patient outcomes in home health care and is now an integral part of the revised *Conditions of Participation* for Medicare-certified home health agencies. OASIS is the result of many years of research, development and demonstration programs funded by CMS and the Robert Wood Johnson Foundation. The current release (OASIS-B1) is a set of 79 items refined by expert panels and demonstration programs. Routine patient assessment approaches are the intended source of information. Among the data items is the fact of death at home.

Data Related to Initiatives for Assessing and Improving the Quality of Care

Two large initiatives aimed at assessing and improving the quality of care provided by health care organizations also warrant consideration: (1)

the ORYX initiative of the Joint Commission on the Accreditation of Healthcare Organizations (JCAHO); and (2) the Health Plan Employer Data and Information Set (HEDIS) of the National Committee for Quality Assurance (NCQA).

JCAHO's ORYX Initiative

JCAHO evaluates and accredits nearly 19,000 health care organizations and programs in the United States. Accreditation by JCAHO is recognized nationwide as an indication that an organization has met certain performance standards. To earn and maintain accreditation, an organization must undergo an on-site survey by a JCAHO survey team at least every three years.

In 1997, JCAHO announced the ORYX initiative, which integrates outcomes and other performance measurement data into the accreditation process. During the current phase of ORYX, accredited agencies collect and submit data on a minimum of six performance measures available through enrollment in any of over 250 listed performance measurements systems.

In May 2001, JCAHO announced four initial core measurement areas for hospitals: acute myocardial infarction, heart failure, community-acquired pneumonia, and pregnancy and related conditions. Hospitals will begin collecting these data for patient discharges beginning July 1, 2002. JCAHO is striving to make core measures for home care and long-term care organizations as consistent as possible with the CMS requirements for OASIS and the nursing home MDS. The ORYX initiative should prove to be a useful source of detailed information about care provided for select conditions relevant to the end of life, but until a significant amount of data become available, its value will not be known.

NCQA's Health Plan Employer Data and Information Set (HEDIS)

NCQA is an independent, non-profit organization whose mission is to evaluate and report on the quality of the nation's managed care organizations. NCQA evaluates health plans against 60 different standards that fall into the following broad categories: access and service, qualified providers, health promotion activities, and quality of care of acute and chronically ill.

NCQA's HEDIS is a tool used by more than 90 percent of health plans to measure performance on important dimensions of care and service. Among the more than 60 measures in HEDIS are measures related to patient satisfaction, inpatient utilization, frequency of selected procedures, and disease-specific treatments such as the use of beta-blockers after a heart attack. The purpose of this data collection is to assist employers and consumers in selecting the best health plan for their needs.

The Quality Compass, a national database of HEDIS and NCQA accreditation information from hundreds of health plans, makes it possible to look at health plans side by side to see how they compare.

TOOLS FOR ACCESSING DATA

Many of the agencies sponsoring large data collection efforts have made useful tools publicly available to facilitate access to the aggregate data. For example, the Federal Electronic Research and Review Extraction Tool (FERRET) is a collaborative effort between the National Center for Health Statistics and the Bureau of the Census to provide full access to complex federally sponsored datasets through the Internet. Currently, the 1994 Underlying Cause-of-Death File, the 1993 NHIS, and NHANES III are available via FERRET, which provides the capabilities to create cross tabulations, frequencies, and SAS or ASCII output files.

CDC Wonder is an easy-to-use system that provides a single point of access to a wide variety of reports, guidelines, and data from the Centers for Disease Control and Prevention. Data can be readily summarized and analyzed from public-use datasets about mortality, cancer incidence, hospital discharges, AIDS, behavioral risk factors, diabetes and many other topics.

The National Center for Health Statistics also maintains the Statistical Export and Tabulation System (SETS), which gives data users the tools to access and manipulate large data files such as the NHIS, LSOA, NHHCS, and NNHS. An example of a more specialized data tool is SEER Stat, which provides cancer investigators with an easy-to-use desktop system for the production of statistics useful in studying the impact of cancer on a population.

In addition to these aggregate-level data tools, data warehouses, such as the National Archive of Computerized Data on Aging (http://www.icpsr.umich.edu/NACDA/index.html) and the National Center for Health Statistics Data Warehouse (http://www.cdc.gov/nchs/datawh.htm), provide means to access the public use data files for many federally sponsored surveys.

INFORMATION MOST READILY AVAILABLE FROM EXISTING DATA SOURCES

Table 3-1 summarizes the types of data available from those datasets presented in this chapter that contain individual-level information. Addi-

tional information about how each dataset captures information in selected categories is found in Appendix B.

LIMITATIONS OF EXISTING DATA SOURCES IN
ANSWERING KEY QUESTIONS

Currently available datasets often provide only sketchy answers to
pressing questions about the end of life among adults. For children, no
reliable answers to these questions emerge from any dataset. The recent
IOM report, *When Children Die* (IOM, 2002), found a similar situation, and
recommends better data collection. (The reader is referred to that report
for more detail.) Examples of the limitations of existing data in answering
the questions listed at the end of Chapter 2 are noted below and comprehensively in Table 3-1.

• *Question #1: Where are people dying and how much of the end of
their lives is spent in those settings?* The site of death is recorded on a
death certificate, but the period of time spent in that final setting is not
noted.

• *Question #2: Who is providing care for them as they die?* Infer-
ences about the use of formal care can be derived from administrative
reimbursement-related data. The National Hospital Discharge Survey
provides an opportunity to look at the subset of discharged deceased to
learn more about patterns among final hospital stays (length of stay, cost,
procedures performed). Little information is available about informal
caregiving. Some health surveys ask community-based respondents questions about assistance with activities of daily living. However, there are
few surveys seeking detailed information directly from care-givers. We
know little about who was available to provide informal care at the end of
life, who actually provided care, and who assisted in the coordination of
care.

• *Question #3: Are physical and psychological symptoms being
identified and treated?* Only 6 of the 16 datasets analyzed included questions about physical symptoms. All 6 asked about pain; 3 also included
questions about shortness of breath, and 2 collected data about fatigue.
Information was obtained about anxiety, depression, or "emotional problems" in 6 datasets. In addition to the presence of symptoms, however,
treatments and procedures directed at ameliorating symptoms are important. The recent increase in inclusion of information about pain in record
keeping by hospitals, home health agencies, hospices and nursing homes
data systems will provide an opportunity to better monitor progress towards reducing pain at the end of life. By allowing us to track the aggregate responses to these questions over time, future data from sources such

as the MDS, OASIS, and JCAHO-mandated records will play a key role in determining if persistent pain is a problem and, if so, whether it is the result of inattention, inadequate treatment, or is simply unavoidable.

• *Question #4: How many persons experience impaired cognitive function before death, to what extent, and for what period of time?* Information about cognitive function is available in nine datasets, though these data are generally cross-sectional. Important information could be gained from the analyses of this information if data points are close in time to the date of death. We know very little about the degree to which cognitive impairment affects communication about dying.

• *Question #5: How many persons experience physical disability or social isolation before death, to what extent, and for what period of time?* Physical disability is captured in 14 of the analyzed datasets, though the structure and wording of questions vary considerably, making comparisons and assessments of change very difficult. Social networks may be inferred from information about living arrangements collected in many datasets, but the perception of social isolation is not measured.

• *Question #6: How do patients and loved ones perceive their quality of life at various time points prior to death?* Information about quality of life is not readily available. Questions were included in the first wave of the AHEAD study, but other surveys and forms of ongoing record keeping do not generally seek this information.

• *Question #7: Are patients and loved ones achieving a sense of life closure in their relationships and spiritually?* Although the importance of closure at the end of life is being increasingly acknowledged, empirical inquiry is at an early stage of development. No approach to asking about life closure or spirituality has been accepted for widespread use at this time.

• *Question #8: Are patients and loved ones involved in decision making about treatment and care options?* Very limited information is available about the existence of advance directive documents in patient records. Essentially no information is widely available that describes the degree to which these are implemented, how often they are overridden, or if providers and patients have had discussions about goals of treatment.

• *Question #9: Are patients and loved ones receiving timely and adequate information on which to base informed decisions?* No questions surveying patients or loved ones about the degree to which they felt adequately informed were identified.

• *Question #10: Are patients and loved ones receiving supportive services from chaplains, therapists, health aides, and other providers?* None of the datasets analyzed provide a framework to create a comprehensive picture of the availability or utilization of support services.

• *Question #11: Are family physical, emotional and financial re-sources being heavily depleted by the care of a dying family member?* Surveys such as the AHEAD study and the National Long-Term Care Survey have the potential to provide information about the depletion of financial resources at the end of life, but little information is being collected about the physical and emotional burdens of caregiving.

• *Question #12: Are loved ones supported through the grieving process?* No population-based information appears to be available about the availability or utilization of bereavement services.

The recommendations in this report are intended to provide initial direction concerning how we might improve the availability and quality of data to better answer these questions.

4

Methodological Issues in the Collection and Use of Data About Dying

End-of-life researchers and others working more broadly with large datasets have identified several methodological issues that require consideration as we look at the use of existing datasets to better understand quality of life and care at the end of life. Small sample sizes are always an obstacle, particularly when using nationally collected health data that are not focused on people who are dying. For adults, with sufficient accumulation of years of data, large enough samples can be assembled for many kinds of analysis of topics related to dying. For children and young adults, however, that is not the case; there have been no studies to date that have focused closely enough on younger people to provide any useful aggregate information about those approaching the end of life. This chapter describes the most pervasive methodologic issues that make end-of-life research difficult. Some of these issues are specific to research on the dying, but many also apply to other areas of health research. Both the specific and the general are included in this chapter, as they apply to research on death and dying.

METHODOLOGICAL ISSUES IDENTIFIED BY END-OF-LIFE RESEARCHERS

End-of-life researchers have described many challenges associated with efforts to monitor quality of life and quality of care at the end of life, as discussed below: (1) obtaining information from the perspectives of the person dying, the person's loved ones, and health providers; (2) coping with variations in the quality of existing data; (3) coping with the difficulties in collecting data from dying people and their loved ones; (4) characterizing the quality of end-of-life care; and (5) defining the period to be considered the "end of life." A more general issue is the lack of standardized terminology in this field. The various conceptual models described in Chapter 2 of this report (which use the original terms, as reported by authors) begin to suggest the variety of language used. The relatively small community of researchers working in this field do interact closely, but should be encouraged to begin converging on a set of defined terms that can then be used in surveys and other types of research to improve comparability among data sets.

• **Obtaining information from varying perspectives.** A full evaluation of the quality of life and quality of care at the end of life requires information from several perspectives: (1) that of the person dying, (2) that of dying person's loved ones who are intimately involved in the person's death, and (3) that of health care providers who are in a unique position to judge the quality of care with respect to current science and professional standards and to report the services used. Most clinicians and researchers acknowledge the importance of the patient's perspective in understanding quality of care, as well as the importance of recognizing the family as the target of care (Donaldson and Field, 1998; Stewart et al., 1999; Teno et al., 1999). Gathering data in a systematic way that captures the perspectives of patients, their loved ones, and health providers is challenging, though—and at present, it is basically not done.

• **Coping with variations in the quality of existing data.** A second challenge is dealing with the variation in quality—i.e., completeness, reliability, and validity—of available data. Information about quality of life and quality of care at the end of life is important to clinicians and to researchers, to individuals and organizations interested in internal quality improvement efforts, and to agencies concerned with external inspections. As this field of inquiry grows and develops, there will be variations in the precision of the data collection and in acceptable standards for reliability and validity. Clearly, some early pilot studies will have to use tools that are not validated, but one aim of that type of research will be to learn about the tools and determine whether they can be used widely. Similarly, as we look to large datasets for information, we must weigh the advantages of developing a portrait using the relatively crude tools that exist, with the risk of being misled by the use of data originally designed for a wholly different purpose.

• **Coping with the difficulties in collecting data from dying people and their loved ones.** A third important challenge is coping with the difficulties of collecting data from dying people and their loved ones.

People who are sick enough to die or struggling to cope with the physical and emotional challenges of caring for a dying loved one are much less likely to be able to respond to surveys or interviews than are people without those burdens. Investigators estimate that one in three dying persons is unable to be interviewed close to death because of somnolence, other cognitive deficits, asthenia, or other medical reasons (Teno et al., 2000). Consequently, missing data and the proportion of proxy responses will present significant challenges to those analyzing these data.

• **Characterizing the quality of end-of-life care.** Yet another challenge is characterizing the quality of end-of-life care. Describing quality involves capturing overuse of medical resources and well as underuse, in addition to documenting poor skills and performance on the part of health care providers (Donaldson and Field, 1998). Judgments in these areas are value laden and must be made with careful consideration of the current evidence base. Nonetheless, research suggests that expert panels can adequately identify the appropriateness and quality of care (Brook et al., 1986; Schuster et al., 1998). Assessing continuity and coordination of care is also important to quality, but, again, methods to do this are very limited at this time.

• **Defining the period to be considered the "end of life."** Defining a period of time to be called the "end of life" is problematic. The changing face of death in this country requires an acknowledgment of the chronic nature of eventually fatal illnesses—such as congestive heart failure and end-stage renal disease—as well as a better understanding of the trajectory of dying from complications associated with dementia and frailty in old age (Lunney et al., 2001; Lynn, 2001; Teno et al., 2000). This suggests that initial information gathering be done tentatively, with a wide net that can be progressively narrowed, as we begin to better understand these various pathways to death.

METHODOLOGICAL ISSUES RELATED TO THE USE OF EXISTING DATASETS

There are several methodological issues associated with the use of large datasets created for purposes other than end-of-life research. These generally stem from the methods and sampling strategies used to collect the data for these datasets.

• **Design and scope of the original study**. If an existing dataset is the result of a specific survey, the usefulness of the data for research on the quality of life and care at the end of life will depend in part on the design and scope of the original study. Information from cross-sectional health surveys of the general population may enhance our understanding of quality of life and care at the end of life if the sample was large enough to allow the identification of a sufficient number of decedents. The National Health Interview Survey, for example, collects information from 30,000 respondents each year. Matching information from this survey to the National Death Index has yielded 54,534 decedents over the period between 1986 and 1994 (Schoeni, 2002), allowing very detailed analyses. However, very few surveys are conducted on such a scale. Data from longitudinal panel studies of the elderly or of others at high risk of death are also valuable, provided that the measurement interval is short and likely to result in data collected close to death.

• **Sampling strategies.** Another important methodological issue in using existing datasets to study quality of life and care at the end of life that warrants attention is the sampling strategies that were used to collect data. Large surveys based on household sampling strategies will have limited value for end-of-life study, because findings cannot be generalized to institutionalized populations and may not fully represent the aging population. Many people at the end of life are elderly and/or chronically ill, and likely to be institutionalized or heavily concentrated in age- or income-restricted housing. List-based sampling strategies, such as the use of Medicare beneficiary roles, better tap these key populations, but they also result in data that cannot be generalized to the full spectrum of the terminally ill population.

• **Unit of analysis.** Careful consideration needs to be given to the *unit of analysis* of existing datasets. Institutional-level data that includes information on individual clients could be an important source of information for end-of-life research. Pooling data from multiple institutions, however, requires careful consideration of the original sampling strategies and timing of data collection.

METHODOLOGICAL ISSUES RELATED TO SURVEY METHODS

Several aspects of survey methods are particularly troublesome for the purpose of studying individuals who are elderly or sick enough to die.

• **Variation in responses among people in different age groups.** Various age groups are known to derive different meaning from the same question, and elderly people are less comfortable than younger people with questions that require drawing comparisons or psychological self-description (Herzog and Rodgers, 1992). Elderly respondents also have difficulty making time tradeoff or utility judgments and completing visual analog scales. Furthermore, age, cognitive ability, and health status affect the likelihood, as well as the quality, of responses to questionnaires and interviews.

• **Reliability and validity of administrative data**. The reliability and validity of administrative data is an additional concern. For example, coding error rates within the Healthcare Cost and Utilization Project's National Inpatient Sample were found to vary widely across states, hospitals within states, geographic location, and hospital characteristics (Berthelsen, 2000). Furthermore, information about comorbidity is seriously underreported (Green and Wintfeld, 1993; Iezzoni et al., 1992), especially for patients with life-threatening disorders (Jencks et al., 1988).

• **Use of proxy respondents**. The use of proxy respondents warrants special attention because of the critical role they play in collecting information about people who are cognitively impaired or too sick to be studied directly, because proxy respondents represent the key source of information after a death has occurred. It is important to understand that these proxies are very likely to have been affected by the decedents dying process and death. They may be asked to report both on their own distress as well as provide information about the decedent. Despite this caution, in general, studies report fairly good agreement between subjects and proxies in many types of assessments. A recent review of clinical studies comparing proxy data with other sources of information for adults (Neumann et al., 2000) found the following:

• Spouses, children, or other close family members tend to be capable proxies, although proxy reports may be influenced by caregiving burden.
• Proxy and subject reports are often comparable in describing levels of functioning, although proxies tend to identify more impairment.
• Proxies and subjects generally agree on overall health, chronic physical conditions, and physical symptoms.
• Relatively little is known about the comparability of proxy reports regarding health care utilization.
• There is low to moderate agreement between proxies and subjects regarding depressive symptoms and psychological well-being, with proxies describing more problems.
• Proxies are often in agreement with subjects on reports of cognitive status, although proxies may overestimate cognitive abilities.

• **Variation in agreement between subjects and proxies.** Variation limits the validity of some data and hampers the comparison of large datasets that contain differing proportions of proxy responses. When possible, it is important to adjust for proxy responses with the development of a predictive model based on a subset of data for which both patient and proxy responses are available for comparison.

• **Difficulties in measuring complex variables.** The measurement of complex variables inevitably introduces another difficult issue—sources of measurement variation among surveys and within rounds of the same survey. The measurement of a person's disability or functional status is a useful example of this issue. First, there are multiple accepted ways of measuring function, including (1) questionnaires or observations of activities of daily living (ADLs) or instrumental activities of daily living (IADLs); (2) questions about physical activity, exercise, or recreation; (3) questions about mobility, range of motion, strength, and endurance; and (4) clinically administered performance batteries. Within just one approach—self-administered questionnaires concerning ADLs—seemingly minor differences in the structure and wording of a questionnaire result in major differences in prevalence estimates of disability (Freedman and Martin, 2000; Picavet and van den Bos, 1996; Wiener et al., 1990). Many of the dimensions of quality at the end of life are equally complex and prone to measurement variation.

ANALYTIC ISSUES IN USING DATA FROM IDENTIFIED DECEDENTS

When using data from identified decedents, important analytic issues arise:

• **Approaches to handling incomplete data.** Handling incomplete data is challenging because variables are likely to be missing for specific reasons, and their absence may bias overall results. Those most in pain or most disabled are perhaps the least likely to provide data points near the end of life. Careful consideration should be given to techniques to reduce non-response biases (Lemke and Drube, 1992).

• **Approaches to describing health and functional status.** Describing the health and functional status of people sick enough to die is especially difficult because of the complexity of the conditions that interact to produce a given state and then change at individually varying rates over time. Multivariate statistical approaches are essential, but even then, careful consideration should be given to capturing individual heterogeneity within complex health states (Manton and Woolson, 1992). This observation implies that subjective, narrative (i.e., expansive) data are needed to supplement the categorical data usually collected in large datasets.

• **Approaches to operationalizing longevity.** Operationalizing longevity has been approached in various ways. The majority of studies take the approach of a direct comparison of decedents with survivors at the end of the follow-up period, but other studies incorporate survival time either through methods that compare sample mortality to population mortality (e.g., Cox proportional hazards model for the statistical analysis of failure time data) or by basing measures on observed mortality (e.g., Palmore's longevity quotient).

• **Addressing the interaction between length of life and outcomes of care.** The interaction of length of life and outcomes of care raises another thorny problem. Most variables relevant to health tend to get "worse" near death; for example, pain, costs of care, caregiver burden, disability. Consequently, care strategies that prolong survival—which themselves may be considered poor outcomes if they only prolong the dying process—may appear to produce poorer outcomes because of the larger numbers of subjects who then fall within this prolonged stage of worsening outcomes. On the other hand, strategies that appear to improve valued outcomes may do so only by shortening lifespan, thus compressing the period of observation during which these negative outcomes tend to be observed.

ISSUES RELATED TO PRIVACY, CONFIDENTIALITY, AND LINKING DATASETS

The idea of linking records, created for different purposes, and possibly at different times and places, of a single individual, is not new. A recent report of the U.S. General Accounting Office (GAO, 2001) cites a paper from the 1950s that discusses linking data from different sources through matching names. Since that time, it has become increasingly clear that linking data sources can create information not available from single sources, and has the potential to reduce both the costs of data collection and the burden on respondents. As part of the effort to "reinvent government," the U.S. Department of Health and Human Services (HHS) has undertaken a major planning effort to restructure its health surveys. Multiple HHS data collection efforts are now linked analytically through the use of common core questionnaires, common sampling frames, and common definitions and terms. This results in an overall reduction in the burden imposed on survey respondents, increases the efficiencies of data collection, and vastly improves the analytic capabilities of HHS surveys (HHS, 1995).

In this report, the value of data linkage is recognized, but the issues related to it are, as well. The committee made no recommendations specifically about privacy issues because, as described in this section, these issues receive a great deal of attention from various public and private entities, which have been working successfully toward both increasing linkages and safeguarding privacy and confidentiality.

Linked records do not raise entirely new privacy issues. They are extensions of the privacy issues that have been and continue to be debated, legislated, and regulated in relation to single data sources. But linkage does raise some additional issues. The GAO (2001) identified five examples:

1. Consent to linkage. In some cases data linkage requires that subjects give consent to the linkage, but in other cases, they may be unaware that, in essence, new information about them is being created. Some linkages require data sharing between agencies, and when this occurs, certain laws and policies concerning disclosure and consent are relevant. Notably, the Privacy Act generally requires consent for disclosure from one agency to another, but there are exceptions.

2. Data sharing. In order to compile the information needed for record linkage and "make the link," agencies must often share identifiable person-specific data. But traditionally, data have been kept separately, and various statutes have been enacted to prohibit or control certain kinds of data sharing. Privacy concerns stem from a desire to control information about oneself and a perceived potential for inappropriate government use (e.g., to pursue criminal charges). Security risks could also arise during data transfer.

3. Reidentification risks. Some datasets are linked using a code-number procedure or are stripped of explicit identifiers as soon after the linkage as possible; nevertheless, reidentification of at least some data subjects may be possible through a deductive process, so only controlled use would be appropriate. To facilitate broader access to statistical and research data, agencies have created more fully "deidentified" public-use datasets (ICDAG, 1999). Although many linked datasets are not made available for public use, some are—and concerns about the reidentification risks associated with these datasets are increasing.

4. Potential sensitivity. The potential sensitivity of data (risk of harm to data subjects) cuts across all other privacy issues. This is true for linked data as well as for single-source datasets. However, linkage may heighten the sensitivity of data that, taken by themselves, appear to be relatively innocuous.

5. Security of linked data. Security is crucial to protecting stored data. For linked data, this is especially true because a linked dataset may be more detailed or more sensitive than its components.

In response to these concerns, and as data linkages have become more common, techniques for protecting privacy and improving "data stewardship" have also developed, through the leadership of various groups, including the Office of Management and Budget and its Interagency Council on Statistical Policy, the Federal Committee on Statistical Methodology, and Confidentiality and Data Access Committee; and the DHHS Data Council[1] and the DHHS Office for Human Research Protections. The National Research Council and its Committee on National Statistics, and the IOM have issue also issued reports dealing with these issues (e.g., NAS, 2000; NCPB, 2000)

Laws and Regulations Affecting Linked Data

The Privacy Act of 1974 establishes governmentwide policies for the disclosure of data by federal agencies and requires agencies to safeguard identifiable information. Under the act, agencies may not disclose identifiable information to third parties without the individual's prior consent. The act contains 12 categories of exceptions to the consent requirement, intended to accommodate legitimate needs for identifiable information, such as conducting research and statistical activities that involve record linkage. In addition, there are certain federal regulations, most notably the Federal Policy for the Protection of Human Subjects, known as the Common Rule, that govern certain research projects that involve human subjects or personal information on them; these projects may include record linkage. Under the Common Rule (HHS regulations codified at part 45, Part 46, Subpart A of the Code of Federal Regulations), research supported or regulated by any of 17 federal agencies is subject to certain federal oversight requirements. In accordance with the Common Rule, organizations have established local institutional review boards (IRBs), made up of both scientists and nonscientists, to approve or disapprove research projects depending on such factors as whether researchers minimize the risks to research subjects and obtain their informed consent.

Tools to Ensure Privacy of Linked Records

GAO (2001) identified the tools relevant to assuring the privacy and confidentiality of linked records, which include:

---

[1]The HHS Data Council consists of HHS officials who have a direct reporting relationship to the Secretary, the HHS Privacy Advocate, and the Senior Advisor on Health Statistics. The Council coordinates HHS data collection and analysis activities, including privacy policy activities.

- techniques for masked data sharing,
- procedures for reducing reidentification risks (including safer data and safer settings), and
- techniques to reduce the sensitivity of the data being linked.

Techniques for masked sharing or linkage include list inflation, third-party models, and grouped linkage. Secure transfer is aided by techniques, such as encryption, as well as physically secure transfer vehicles (e.g., secure data lines). Safeguard reviews can help ensure that security measures are being followed in another agency. Obtaining consent or providing the ability to "opt out" may be necessary for at least some linkage projects. One approach, used in the Health and Retirement Study, is an explicit consent form, which asks the respondent's permission for specific records to be transferred from SSA to the University of Michigan for the purpose of linkage. The basic physical and electronic security approaches that are used to protect any data stored electronically also are relevant for information resulting from record linkage. These include access controls, audit trails, and storage strategies. (NRC, 1997; IRS, 2000; Jabine, 1993; GAO, 2001b; 2000a,b,c; 1999; 1998). Stewardship involves compliance with relevant laws as well as the coordination of project-by-project decisions, (which may include whether or not to conduct a specific linkage or whether to release linked data); systems for accountability; and organizational culture.

5

Conclusions and Recommendations

In order to better understand how Americans die and to improve the care received by those at the end of life, we must look beyond the death itself to the experience of chronic and terminal illness as well as dying and bereavement. The prevention of premature death will always be a key public health goal, but the well-being of the nation will also be served by the prevention of unnecessary suffering at life's end. A better description of how Americans of all ages currently die and the impact on their families is much needed and must be followed by continuing efforts to track changes over time. Both the quality of dying and the quality of the health care provided at the end of life should be addressed.

No single type of data collection will provide the full range of information needed to comprehensively describe the quality of life and quality of care at the end of life. And the broad sweeps that are the focus of this report should be associated with small focused studies to better understand patterns—such as geographic variation—that can be *detected* at the national level, but only *understood* at the local level. Longitudinal, population-based panels will continue to provide an important opportunity to observe events that may have significance to dying when death cannot be predicted. A nationally representative follow-back survey of the next of kin of decedents is essential to capture the depth of information needed to adequately describe events immediately surrounding death. And, finally, surveys of health care agencies and providers are needed to collect information on quality of care from the professional.

Recommendations to make the best use of current data collection efforts as well as fill important gaps address three broad questions:

- What could be learned from already existing data?
- What modifications would improve the usefulness of currently collected data?
- What new steps should be taken to enhance the accuracy and richness of data collection to better monitor and improve the quality of life and care at the end of life for patients of all ages and their affected families?

Recommendation #1:
Support Researchers' Use of Existing Data Systems

Agencies should promote research that uses existing data resources to describe aspects of the quality of life and quality of care at the end of life, by publicizing their availability and providing funding for analysis.

A great deal of information is recorded, for a variety of purposes, that could describe aspects of quality of life and quality of care at the end of life. It is probably not surprising that Medicare claims and other data collected for purposes other than measuring quality at the end of life are not always used to their fullest for measuring quality, given that their primary purpose is purely administrative. In addition, the full potential value of many surveys and studies of health and well-being in characterizing quality of life and care at the end of life is not realized because data are analyzed only to answer some questions but not others. The reasons for this vary, but include a general lack of funding support for further data analysis, the fact that researchers are unaware of the data resource, and in some cases, the relatively new ability to link data from different sources to facilitate meaningful answers to important questions.

Currently, little support is available to researchers to make use of existing data resources in describing aspects of the quality of life and and the care provided to individuals who are dying. Research-funding agencies should provide support for using existing data resources for this purpose. Some examples of the types of studies that could be conducted with modest funding include:

- Making use of existing longitudinal surveys to examine the health trajectories of those who die in order to learn more about the role of suffering, disability, and chronic illnesses at the end of life.
- Studying patterns of costs and utilization in the years before death

to more fully describe the use of home care, hospice care, in-home privately paid help, and informal care.

• Studying the number of care transitions in the last year of life, both in terms of settings and of providers.

• Comparing data from multiple settings with regard to the rates of pain and other symptom assessment, and use of opioids and other symptom-relieving interventions.

• Developing valid indicators of variables and constructs that are important to good end-of-life care. This is an important but slow process—and one that needs to be attended to immediately.

• Examining individual and institutional factors that influence racial and geographic variations in patterns of end-of-life care.

Recommendation #2:
Improve the Usefulness of Existing Data Systems

Government and private organizations should institute training initiatives and make incremental changes to surveys to improve the usefulness of currently collected data in describing aspects of quality of life and quality of care at the end of life.

Training for researchers and incremental changes to surveys would be relatively inexpensive ways to improve the usefulness of currently collected data in describing aspects of quality of life and quality of care at the end of life.

Training for Researchers

More funding for analysis and better publicity about data sources will improve the use of existing information up to a point, but beyond that, researchers may need training in specific datasets or enhancement of skills to be able to understand the possibilities of existing information collection. Focused training opportunities, limited in scope, can open the way for much better use of what data currently exist. Specific recommendations for training of researchers are as follows:

• Government agencies that sponsor data collection should sponsor a series of training initiatives to open dialogues among researchers and health care workers to increase the reliability and validity of ongoing data collections. These should emphasize:

• Training professionals in various disciplines in the use of data sources.

- Training existing palliative care researchers to incorporate research questions in their studies, which would utilize existing data bases.
- Promoting existing health service researchers with expertise in these databases to collaborate with palliative care researchers.

Improving the Quality of Data Recorded

- Professional organizations should promote increased standardization of language through open dialogue about terms that now have diverse meanings, e.g., hospice care, palliative care, and end of life.
- In settings where physicians complete death certificates regularly, institute training and quality control measures.
- The federal government should mandate that institutions and organizations providing care (hospitals, nursing homes, home health agencies, outpatient settings) conduct ongoing quality improvement efforts, including training in recording required data.

Incremental Changes to Ongoing Data Collection Efforts

The information content for studying end-of-life issues can be enhanced in specific surveys by relatively minor changes. The following improvements, modifications, or supplements to ongoing data collection efforts would be relatively inexpensive ways to build upon existing efforts:

- Sponsors of longitudinal health surveys should insist on the routine use of "exit" surveys to capture information from the next-of-kin of participants who die between survey rounds. These supplemental surveys not only enhance the existing survey by covering a more inclusive range of outcomes but can provide rich data about end-of-life issues at relatively low cost.
- Improvements to the information infrastructure, such as nationwide electronic reporting of death certificates, should be made to facilitate more timely collection and analysis of vital information.
- Sampling frames for current surveys should be carefully reviewed for adequacy both in terms of contemporary housing arrangements and changing health care organizational structures.
- Survey questions regarding health care utilization should include probes that capture need for and use of the full range of supportive services.
- Mechanisms should be put in place for continuous refinement of large ongoing surveys, using input from a wide variety of sources. Web-

based opportunities to e-mail questions and suggestions would facilitate this exchange.

• The Centers for Medicare and Medicaid Services (CMS)—formerly known as the Health Care Financing Administration—should consider minor increases in the data elements recorded on Medicare claims under the hospice benefit. This topic should be addressed by the Medicare Payment Advisory Commission (MedPAC), a Congressionally-mandated organization that advises CMS on the Medicare system. Ongoing efforts should be directed towards facilitating links among key types of data collection, especially between surveys and health care utilization records.

Recommendation #3:
A New National Mortality Followback Survey

The federal government should undertake a new National Mortality Followback Survey to enhance the accuracy and richness of data collection related to quality of life and care at the end of life.

A new National Mortality Followback Survey program of regular, periodic surveys that gather comparable data over time, should be initiated. The new NMFS would be a collaborative effort between the National Center for Health Statistics (which would carry out the survey), the National Institutes of Health (NIH), and the Agency for Healthcare Research and Quality (the latter organizations would sponsor the survey). As the lead institute for end-of-life research at the NIH, the National Institute of Nursing Research could take a major role in supporting a National Mortality Followback Survey and determining content, with collaboration from other NIH institutes (in particular, the National Institute on Aging, but possibly including some of the disease-oriented institutes), and the Agency for Healthcare Research and Quality. Three specific aims should be considered for future National Mortality Followback Surveys. First, a major focus should be on determining the extent of morbidity experienced at the end of life, to aid the long-range goal of reducing unnecessary morbidity. Second, deaths among children should be over-sampled in order to yield information specific to this understudied group. And third, minority populations should be over-sampled to improve understanding of ethnic and racial differences in the experience of death and dying in the United States.

References

Arnett R. Health Services Data Sources in the U.S. In: Armitage P, Colton T, editors. Encyclopedia of Biostatistics. New York: John Wiley, 1998: 1869-1877.

Backlund E, Sorlie PD, Johnson NJ. A comparison of the relationships of education and income with mortality: The National Longitudinal Mortality Study. Soc Sci Med 1999; 49(10):1373-1384.

Berthelsen CL. Evaluation of coding data quality of the HCUP National Inpatient Sample. Top Health Inf Manage 2000; 21(2):10-23.

Brook RH, Chassin MR, Fink A, Solomon DH, Kosecoff J, Park RE. A method for the detailed assessment of the appropriateness of medical technologies. Int J Technol Assess Health Care 1986; 2(1):53-63.

Christakis NA, Escarce JJ. Survival of Medicare patients after enrollment in hospice programs. N Engl J Med 1996; 335:172-178.

Christakis NA, Iwashyna TJ. Impact of individual and market factors on the timing of initiation of hospice terminal care. Med Care 2000; 38(5):528-41.

Donaldson MS, Field MJ. Measuring quality of care at the end of life. Arch Intern Med 1998; 158(2):121-128.

Emanuel EJ, Emanuel LL. The promise of a good death. Lancet 1998; 351 Suppl 2:SII21-SII29.

Freedman VA, Martin LG. Contribution of chronic conditions to aggregate changes in old-age functioning. Am J Public Health 2000; 90(11):1755-1760.

Green J, Wintfeld N. How accurate are hospital discharge data for evaluating effectiveness of care? Med Care 1993; 31(8):719-731.

Hawes C, Morris JN, Phillips CD, Mor V, Fries BE, Nonemaker S. Reliability estimates for the Minimum Data Set (MDS) for nursing home resident assessment and care screening. Gerontologist 1995; 35(2):172-178.

HCFA. Memorandum on Minimum Data Set State Operations Manual. Health Care Financing Administration. 9-2-1998 (CMS Web site).

Herzog AR, Rodgers WL. The use of survey methods in research on older Americans. In: Wallace RB, Woolson RF, editors. The Epidemiologic Study of the Elderly. New York: Oxford University Press, 1992: 60-90.

HHS. HHS Plan for Integration of Surveys. Department of Health and Human Services. 4-11-1995 (Web site).

HHS. Standards for Privacy of Individually Identifiable Health Information. Office for Civil Rights. 4-14-2001. 11-28-2001 (Web site).

Hogan C, Lunney J, Gabel J, Lynn J. Medicare beneficiaries' costs of care in the last year of life. Health Affairs 2001; 20(4):188-195.

Hogan C, Lynn J, Gabel J, Lunney J, O'Mara A, Wilkinson A. A statistical profile of decedents in the Medicare program. 00-1. 3-7-2000. Medicare Payment Advisory Commission. Contractor Research Series.

Iezzoni LI, Foley SM, Daley J, Hughes J, Fisher ES, Heeren T. Comorbidities, complications, and coding bias. Does the number of diagnosis codes matter in predicting in-hospital mortality? JAMA 1992; 267(16):2197-2203.

Institute of Medicine. Approaching Death: Improving Care at the End of Life. Field MJ, Cassel CK, editors. Washington, DC: National Academy Press, 1997.

Institute of Medicine. Ensuring Quality Cancer Care. Hewitt M, Simone JV, eds. Washington, DC: National Academy Press, 1999.

Institute of Medicine. Improving Palliative Care for Cancer. Foley KM, Gelband H, eds. Washington, DC: National Academy Press, 2001.

Institute of Medicine. When Children Die: Improving Palliative and End-of-life Care for Children and Their Families. Field MJ, Behrman RE, editors. Washington, DC: The National Academies Press, 2002.

Interagency Confidentiality and Data Access Group. "Checklist on Disclosure Potential of Proposed Data Releases." Washington, DC: OMB Federal Committee on Statistical Methodology, July 1999.

Internal Revenue Service. Tax Information Security Guidelines for Federal, State, and Local Agencies: Safeguards for Protecting Federal Tax Returns and Return Information (Pub. 1075). Washington, DC: June 2000. Available at ftp://ftp.fedworld.gov/pub/irs-utl/pub1075.pdf.

Jabine TB. "Procedures for Restricted Data Access." Journal of Official Statistics 1993; 9(2):537-589.

Jencks SF, Williams DK, Kay TL. Assessing hospital-associated deaths from discharge data. The role of length of stay and comorbidities. JAMA 1988; 260(15):2240-2246.

Johnson NJ, Backlund E, Sorlie PD, Loveless CA. Marital status and mortality: The national longitudinal mortality study. Ann Epidemiol 2000; 10(4):224-238.

Kaufman JS, Kaufman S. Assessment of structured socioeconomic effects on health. Epidemiology 2001; 12(2):157-167.

Lemke JH, Drube GA. Issues in Handling Incomplete Data in Surveys of the Elderly. In: Wallace RB, Woolson RF, editors. The Epidemiologic Study of the Elderly. New York: Oxford University Press, 1992: 358-369.

Lilienfeld A, Lilienfield D. Foundations of Epidemiology. 2nd ed. New York: Oxford University Press, 1980.

Lloyd-Jones DM, Martin DO, Larson MG, Levy D. Accuracy of death certificates for coding coronary heart disease as the cause of death. Ann Intern Med 1998; 129(12):1020-1026.

Lunney JR, Lynn J, Hogan C. Profiles of Elderly Medicare Decedents. 2001. (unpublished)

Lynn J. Measuring quality of care at the end of life: A statement of principles. J Am Geriatr Soc 1997; 45:526-527.

Lynn J. Perspectives on care at the close of life. Serving patients who may die soon and their families: the role of hospice and other services. JAMA 2001; 285(7):925-932.

Manton KG, Woolson R. Grade of Membership Analysis in the Epidemiology of Aging. In: Wallace RB, Woolson RF, editors. The Epidemiologic Study of the Elderly. New York: Oxford University Press, 1992: 333-357.

Maudsley G, Williams EM. Inaccuracy in death certification—where are we now? J Public Health Med 1996; 18(1):59-66.

Minino AM, Smith BL. Deaths: Preliminary data for 2000. National vital statistics reports, vol. 49, no. 12. Hyattsville, MD: National Center for Health Statistics 2001.

National Cancer Institute (NCI). SEER Web site. http://SEER.cancer.gov. Accessed April 26, 2002.

National Cancer Policy Board, Institute of Medicine, and National Research Council. Enhancing Data Systems to Improve the Quality of Cancer Care. Hewitt M, Simone JV, editors. Washington, DC: National Academy Press, 2000.

National Research Council. For the Record: Protecting Electronic Health Information. Washington, DC: National Academy Press, 1997.

National Research Council, Committee on National Statistics, Commission on Behavioral and Social Sciences and Education. Improving Access to and Confidentiality of Research Data: Report of a Workshop. Mackie C, Bradburn N, editors. Washington, DC: National Academy Press, 2000.

Nerenz DR. Capacities and limitations of information systems as data sources on quality of care at the end of life. J Pain Symptom Manage 2001; 22(3):773-783.

Neumann PJ, Araki SS, Gutterman EM. The use of proxy respondents in studies of older adults: Lessons, challenges, and opportunities. J Am Geriatr Soc 2000; 48(12):1646-1654.

Panel on Confidentiality and Data Access. Private Lives and Public Policies. Washington, DC: National Academy Press, 1993.

Paul JE, Weis KA, Epstein RA. Data bases for variations research. Med Care 1993; 31(5 Suppl):YS96-102.

Picavet HS, van den Bos GA. Comparing survey data on functional disability: The impact of some methodological differences. J Epidemiol Community Health 1996; 50(1):86-93.

Ries LAG, Eisner, MP, Kosary CL, Hankey BF, Miller BA, Clegg LX, Edwards BK, editors. SEER Cancer Statistics Review, 1973-1997, National Cancer Institute. NIH Pub. No. 00-2789. Bethesda, MD: 2000.

Riley G, Lubitz J, Prihoda R, Rabey E. The use and costs of Medicare services because of death. Inquiry 1987; 24(3):233-244.

Riley GF, Potosky AL, Lubitz JD, Kessler LG. Medicare payments from diagnosisto death for elderly cancer patients by stage at diagnosis. Med Care 1995; 33(8):828-841.

Schoeni RF, Freedman V, Wallace RB. Late-Life Disability Trajectories and Socioeconomic Status. 2002 (unpublished).

Schuster MA, McGlynn EA, Brook RH. How good is the quality of health care in the United States? Milbank Q 1998; 76(4):517-563, 509.

Seeman I, Poe GS, McLaughlin JK. Design of the 1986 National Mortality Followback Survey: Considerations on collecting data on decedents. Pub Health Rep 1989; 104(2):183-188.

Smith Sehdev AE, Hutchins GM. Problems with proper completion and accuracy of the cause-of-death statement. Arch Intern Med 2001; 161(2):277-284.

Steinhauser KE, Christakis NA, Clipp EC, McNeilly M, McIntyre L, Tulsky JA. Factors considered important at the end of life by patients, family, physicians, and other care providers. JAMA 2000a; 284(19):2476-2482.

Steinhauser KE, Clipp EC, McNeilly M, Christakis NA, McIntyre LM, Tulsky JA. In search of a good death: Observations of patients, families, and providers. Ann Intern Med 2000b; 132(10):825-832.

Stewart AL, Teno J, Patrick DL, Lynn J. The concept of quality of life of dying persons in the context of health care. J Pain Symptom Manage 1999; 17(2):93-108.

Teno JM, Byock I, Field MJ. Research agenda for developing measures to examine quality of care and quality of life of patients diagnosed with life-limiting illness. J Pain Symptom Manage 1999; 17(2):75-82.

Teno JM, Fisher E, Hamel MB, Wu AW, Murphy DJ, Wenger NS et al. Decision-making and outcomes of prolonged ICU stays in seriously ill patients. J Am Geriatr Soc 2000; 48(5 Suppl):S70-S74.

Teno JM, McNiff K, Lynn J. Measuring Quality of Medical Care for Dying Persons and Their Families. In: Lawton MP, editor. Annu Rev Gerontol Geriatr. New York: Springer, 2001: 97-119.

Teno JM. Quality of care and quality indicators for lives ended by cancer. In: Foley KM, Gelband H, editors. Improving Palliative Care for Cancer. Washington, DC: National Academy Press, 2001.

U.S. General Accounting Office. Record linkage and privacy: Issues in creating new federal research and statistical information. GAO-01-126SP, 2001a.

U.S. General Accounting Office. High risk series: An update. GAO-01-263, 2001b.

U.S. General Accounting Office. Computer security: Critical federal operations and assets remain at risk. GAO/T-AIMD-00-314, 2000a.

U.S. General Accounting Office. Information security: Serious and widespread weaknesses persist at federal agencies. GAO/AIMD-00-295, 2000b.

U.S. General Accounting Office. Medicare: Improvements needed to enhance protection of confidential health information. GAO/HEHS-99-140, July 29, 1999.

U.S. General Accounting Office. Information security: Serious weaknesses place critical federal operations and assets at risk. GAO/AIMD-98-92, Sept. 23, 1998.

Virnig BA, Fisher ES, McBean AM, Kind S. Hospice use in Medicare managed care and fee-for-service systems. Am J Managed Care 2001; 7:777-786.

Virnig BA, Kind S, McBean, AM, Fisher ES. Geographic variation in hospice use prior to death. J Am Geriatrics Soc 2000; 48:1117-1125.

Virnig BA, McBean AM, Kind S, Dholakia R. Hospice use prior to death: Variability across cancer diagnoses. Med Care 2002; 40:73-78.

Virnig BA, Morgan RO, Persily NA, DeVito CA. Racial and income differences in use of the Medicare hospice benefit between the HMO and FFS systems. J Palliative Med 1999a; 2(1):23-31.

Virnig BA, Persily NA, Morgan RO, DeVito CA. Do Medicare HMOs and Medicare FFS differ in their use of the Medicare hospice benefit? Hospice J 1999b; 14:1-12.

Weeks J. Personal communication. 10-2-2001.

Wiener JM, Hanley RJ, Clark R, Van Nostrand JF. Measuring the activities of daily living: Comparisons across national surveys. J Gerontol 1990; 45(6):S229-S237.

Wolinsky FD, Stump TE, Johnson RJ. Hospital utilization profiles among older adults over time: Consistency and volume among survivors and decedents. J Gerontol B Psychol Sci Soc Sci 1995; 50(2):S88-100.

Appendix A

Administrative Information for Relevant Datasets

ADMINISTRATIVE INFORMATION

dataset	Health and Retirement Study	**abbrev**	HRS
parent study			

first year	1992	**last year**	2000
sponsor	NIA		
collector	Institute for Social Research, University of Michigan		
PI	Robert J. Willis		

purpose to explain the antecedents and consequences of retirement; to examine the relationship between health, income, and wealth over time; to examine life cycle patterns of wealth accumulation and consumption; to monitor work disability; and to examine how the mix and distribution of economic, family and program resources affect key outcomes, including retirement, savings, health declines and institutionalization

topics health and cognitive conditions, status; retirement plans and perspectives; attitudes, preferences, expectations, and subjective probabilities; family structure and transfers; employment status and job history; job demands and requirements; disability, demographic background, housing, income and net worth, health insurance and pension plans

design   national panel study

baseline   in home, face-to-face in 1992 for the 1931-1941 birth cohort and in 1998 for newly added 1924-1930 and 1942-1947 birth cohorts

followup   follow-ups by telephone every second year, with proxy interviews after death

design notes   merged with AHEAD in 1998

sample   12,600 persons in 7,600 households   **% proxy**

sample notes   100% oversamples of Hispanics, Blacks, and Florida residents

number of decedents

questionnaire available **coding information available**   **bibliography**

links   Employer Pension Study (1993, 1999); National Death Index, Social Security Administration

availability of data publicly available data on www.umich.edu/~hrswww includes HRS Wave 1,2,3 (soon 4)

contacts

ADMINISTRATIVE INFORMATION

dataset   Longitudinal Study of Aging   **abbrev** LSOA

parent study   National Health Interview Survey (NHIS) 1984 Supplement on Aging

first year   1984   **last year**   1990

sponsor

collector	**PI**
purpose	to measure transitions in functional status and living arrangements for a national representative cohort of Americans who were aged 70 and older in 1984 and lived in the community; a second survey was field on a cohort derived from the 1994 NHIS
topics	functioning, family structure, housing and living arrangements, health care, economic and retirement indicators, vital status
design	longitudinal panel
baseline	1984 baseline personal interviews called the Supplement on Aging (SOA) were conducted with 16,148 subjects; The LSOA followed 7,527 of these subjects who were 70+
followup	LSOA reinterviews in 1986 (5,151), 1988 (7,541), 1990 (5,978); LSOA II reinterviews were conducted in 1997-1998 and 1999-2000
design notes	used personal interviews in 1984; telephone interviews and mailed questionnaires in 1986-1990; plus record linkage
sample	7,527 **% proxy** 8.5%
sample notes	the LSOA followed those participants in the Supplement on Aging (SOA) to the 1984 NHIS who were 70 years of age and over. The SOA was a systematic one-half sample of people 55-64 in the 1984 NHIS and all people 65+; In 1986, the LSOA interviewed all SOA households with participants 80+; all households with Hispanic or black persons and their relatives 70-79; and half of households with whites aged 70-79. In 1988 and 1990, all participants; The LSOA II used the same methodology
number of decedents	
questionnaire available	**coding information available** **bibliography**
links	National Death Index and Medicare administrative records

availability of data

contacts

ADMINISTRATIVE INFORMATION

dataset   National Mortality Followback Survey   **abbrev** NMFS

parent study

first year   1961   **last year**   1993

sponsor   National Center for Health Statistics

collector   NCHS   **PI**

purpose   to supplement information from death certificates in the vital statistics file with information on important characteristics of the decedent which affect mortality. Objectives vary with each survey round

topics   include use of health services prior to death, socioeconomic status, aspects of life style, health care utilization prior to death, and other factors that affect when and how death occurs; 1993 topics: demographics, SES, manner of death, firearm related injury, motor vehicle/driving behavior, problem behaviors, use of alcohol, drugs, and tobacco, medical examiner/coroner abstract file

design   multicomponent stratified list-based survey

baseline   one time survey of next of kin, with linked data obtained from health care facilities used in the last year of life

followup   n/a

design notes complexity of questionnaire necessitated telephone or in person interviews; 83% response rate; 1,000 items focused in 23 domains

sample   22,957   **% proxy**   100%

sample notes drawn from 1993 Current Mortality Sample (10% systematic random sample of death certificates): sampling strata: age, race, gender, and cause of death; 45% of sample selected with certainty; oversampling of blacks, females, decedents under age 35 and over age 99 (South Dakota declined to participate)

number of 22,957
decedents

questionnaire **coding information** **bibliography**
available **available**

links

availability of data tapes can be purchased through NTIS: four linked
data data files (death certificate file; proxy respondent survey questionnaire; nursing home, hospital, and hospice questionnaire; and facility abstract record)

contacts Mortality Statistics Branch, NCHS, Hyattsville, MD (301)458-4666

ADMINISTRATIVE INFORMATION

dataset National Health and Nutrition Examination

abbrev NHANES

parent study

first year 1960 **last year** ongoing

sponsor NCHS

collector NCHS **PI** Dr. Raynard Kington

purpose to assess the health and nutritional status of adults and children in the United States; to estimate disease prevalence, awareness, treatment and control; to monitor trends in risk behaviors; to study the relationship between diet, nutrition, and health; to establish a national probability sample of genetic material

topics demographics, acculturation, SES and education; diet, dietary supplements, and food security; medical conditions, health care utilization, health insurance and prescription drugs used; physical activity, fitness and function; alcohol, drug, and tobacco use; pesticide use;

includes medical examination and special substudy collecting hair

design annual survey

baseline "snapshot" only, but now linked to Medicare and NDI for longitudinal and historical purposes

followup linked to the NDI and Medicare

design notes now linked to the NHIS at the Primary Sampling Unit (PSU); linked to NHIS with regard to questionnaire content; household screening interview; detailed household interview, individual physical exam and health and dietary interviews in mobile examination centers (or at home if necessary)

sample approx 6,000 per year (5,000 with PE)   **% proxy**

sample notes now each year's data are representative

number of decedents link to NDI; passive mortality study 1976-1980; cohort followup study (NHEFS)

questionnaire available **coding information available** **bibliography**

links National Death Index, Medicare

availability of data data can be ordered from NCHS or downloaded from Web (lag time there)

contacts Raynard Kington, Director NHANES, NCHS, 6525 Belcrest Road, Room 1000, Hyattsville, MD 20782

ADMINISTRATIVE INFORMATION

dataset Medical Expenditure Panel Survey   **abbrev** MEPS

parent study National Medical Care Expenditure Survey (NMCES or NMES)

first year 1977   **last year**   ongoing

sponsor AHRQ & NCHS

collector PI

purpose	provide comprehensive data that estimate the level and distribution of health care use and expenditures, monitor the dynamics of the health care delivery and insurance systems, and assess health care policy implications
topics	health care use, expenditures, sources of payment, insurance coverage, health care status, and disability
design	overlapping panel design
baseline	
followup	
design notes	First two surveys (1977 and 1987) were studies of 14,500 households; 1996 (n = 10,000 households) changed to begin phase in of overlapping panel; will evolve to be 4,000 households brought in each year and followed for 2 years (so 10,000 households in any 2 1/2 year frame)

sample 10,000 households **% proxy**

sample notes linked to NHIS PSU

number of decedents

questionnaire available **coding information available** **bibliography**

links linked to NHIS

availability of data PUFS on Web

contacts MEPSPD@ahrq.gov

ADMINISTRATIVE INFORMATION

dataset Panel Study of Income Dynamics **abbrev** PSID

parent study

first year 1968 **last year** 2001

sponsor NIA, NSF, DHHS/ASPE

collector University of Michigan Institute for Social Research
        PI Sandra Hofferth and Frank Russell

purpose   to provide economic and demographic data at the family and individual level, as well as household

topics   income sources and amounts, employment, family composition changes, childbirth and marriage histories, and residential location; NIA funded supplement on health; some sociological and psychological data in some waves

design   every other year interview

baseline   Initial sample = 2,930 households and 1,872 low income families; households formed by earlier panel members are included in subsequent waves; 1996 sample = 8,885 then reduced by suspending some low income and added new post-1968 immigrant sample

followup   annual interviews conducted 1968-1997; every other year interviewing began 1999

design notes   long-term cumulative response rate was approximately 60% as of 1994

sample   8,895 households in 1997
% proxy   head of household interviewed

sample notes

**number of
decedents**

questionnaire   coding information   bibliography
available   available

links

availability of   main data files updated with each wave;
data   www.umich.edu/~psid

contacts

ADMINISTRATIVE INFORMATION

dataset   Outcome and Assessment Information Set

abbrev   OASIS

parent study

first year   2000   **last year**

sponsor   Center for Medicare and Medicaid Services

collector   agencies submit to CMS   **PI**

purpose   form the core set of data items of a comprehensive assessment of an adult home care patient and form the basis for measuring patient outcomes for purposes of quality improvement

topics   demographics, finances, current illness, therapies, living arrangements, physical assessments, symptoms, function

design   longitudinal

baseline   start of care assessment

followup   follow-up assessment

design notes   either incorporated into agency's data collection forms or can be stand alone data collection

sample   **% proxy**

sample notes

number of decedents

questionnaire available   **coding information available**   **bibliography**

links

availability of data

contacts

ADMINISTRATIVE INFORMATION

dataset   Nursing Home Minimum Data Set (Resident)

abbrev   MDS

parent study   IOM Committee on Nursing Home Regulation

first year   1990   **last year**   ongoing

sponsor   CMS (formerly HCFA)

collector   each agency   **PI**

purpose   to provide a comprehensive assessment of nursing home residents in a standardized format to transmit to HCFA

topics   demographics, customary routine, cognitive patterns, comunication, mood and behavior, physical functioning, continence, disease, nutrition, medications, procedures, therapy

design   longitudinal

baseline   on admission

followup   quarterly or with significant change in status

design notes   research indicates that staff can produce research-quality data, but in practice facilities differ in their commitment to ensuring that staff are trained and adhere to assessment protocols

sample   **% proxy**

sample notes   all nursing home residents

number of decedents   can be identified by discharge assessment

questionnaire available   **coding information available**   **bibliography**

links

availability of data

contacts

ADMINISTRATIVE INFORMATION

dataset   Surveillance, Edpidemiology, and End Results Program

abbrev   SEER

parent study

first year   1973   **last year**   ongoing

sponsor   National Cancer Institute

collector   PI

purpose   to provide information on cancer incidence and survival in the United States

topics   patient demographics, primary tumor site, morphology, stage at diagnosis, first course of treatment, and follow-up for vital status

design   registry of all tumors reported in a geographic area

baseline   standard for case ascertainment is 98%

followup

design notes   in additon to registry information, there is an ongoing program of special studies that collect information through surveys, interviews, record abstraction, and biological materials

sample   14% of U.S. population **% proxy**

sample notes   geographic areas were selected for inclusion based on their ability to operate and maintain a high quality reporting system

**number of
decedents**

questionnaire   coding information   bibliography
available   available

links

availability of   updated annually and provided in print and electronic
data   formats

contacts

ADMINISTRATIVE INFORMATION

dataset   National Home and Hospice Care Survey

abbrev   NHHCS

parent study National Health Care Survey

first year   1992   **last year**   1998

sponsor	NCHS
collector	**PI**
purpose	to document the availability and utilization of home and hospice care
topics	agency characteristics: ownership, affiliation, geographic region, location, certification status; Patient characteristics: age, race, marital status, living arrangements, caregiver status, services received, service providers, reason for discharge
design	cross-sectional survey
baseline	
followup	
design notes	data collected through personal interviews with administrators and staff
sample	16,500 agencies (1998) **% proxy**
sample notes	Stratified, two stage probability design (agency type, MSA, region, ownership, certification) In 1996, 13,500 agencies provided services to 2,486,800 patients, with 8,168,900 discharges; in 1996, 1,800 agencies provided hospice care to 59,400 current patients and had 393,200 discharges (322,200 or 82% = deaths)
number of decedents	1996: 322,200

questionnaire available   **coding information available**   **bibliography**

links	can be linked to OASIS
availability of data	public use data files available through 1998
contacts	Dr. Barbara Haupt

ADMINISTRATIVE INFORMATION

dataset	National Nursing Home Survey	**abbrev** NNHS
parent study	National Health Care Survey	

first year   1973   **last year**   1999

sponsor   NCHS

collector   **PI**

purpose   provide information on nursing homes from the perspec-
                     tive of the provider of services and from the recipient

topics   facilities: size, ownership, certification, occupancy rate,
                     number of days of care provided, expenses; residents:
                     demographic characteristics, health status, and services
                     received

design   cross-sectional survey

baseline   1973-1974, 1977, 1985, 1995, 1997, 1999; consist of facility
                     files, discharge files, resident files, and staff files

followup

design notes   data obtained through personal interviews with adminis-
                     trators and staff (note: information about residents pro-
                     vided by staff member familiar with care provided to
                     resident)

sample   1,500 facilities   **% proxy**

sample notes   up to six current residents and up to six charges are se-
                     lected for individual level interviews

**number of
decedents**

**questionnaire   coding information   bibliography
available   available**

links

availability of public use data files
data

contacts

ADMINISTRATIVE INFORMATION

dataset   National Hospital Discharge Survey   **abbrev** NHDS

parent study   National Health Care Survey

first year 1965 **last year** annually

sponsor NCHS

collector **PI**

purpose provide information on the characteristics of inpatients discharged from non-federal short-stay hospitals

topics age, sex, race, ethnicity, marital status, expected sources of payment, admission and discharge dates, discharge status

design

baseline

followup

design notes note: cannot use individual level data because individuals could have multiple discharges in one year and thus be sampled more than once.

sample 500 hospitals and 270,000 inpatient beds **% proxy**

sample notes Excludes federal, military, VA, prison hospitals, and hospitals with fewer than six beds. All hospitals with 1,000 or more beds are sampled with certainty. Non-certain hospitals selected randomly from PSU sampling units of NHIS

number of decedents in 1996, deaths accounted for 3% of discharges

questionnaire available **coding information available** **bibliography**

links

availability of data electronic files from FTP server

contacts

ADMINISTRATIVE INFORMATION

dataset Healthcare Cost and Utilization Project **abbrev** HCUP

parent study

first year 1988 **last year**

sponsor Agency for Healthcare Research and Quality

collector **PI**

purpose to build a multi-state health care data system about discharges from hospital

topics primary and secondary diagnoses, primary and secondary procedures, admission and discharge status, demographics, expected payment source, total charges, length of stay

design coordinated all payer databases

baseline

followup

design notes

sample 7 million hospital stays **% proxy**

sample notes 22 states participate, approximating a 20% stratified sample of U.S. community hospitals. National Inpatient Sample = 1,000 hospitals

number of decedents

questionnaire **coding information** **bibliography**
available **available**

links

availability of data

contacts

ADMINISTRATIVE INFORMATION

dataset National Vital Statistics Death Certificates

abbrev NVS

parent study

first year 1930 **last year** 1998

sponsor National Center for Health Statistics

collector   NCHS, CDC   **PI**

purpose   to provide national mortality statistics

topics   immediate cause of death, intermediate cause of death, underlying cause of death, other coexisting conditions; age, race, marital status, educational attainment, occupation

design   continuous reporting by states to Bureau of Census

baseline

followup

design notes

sample   2.3 million in 1998   **% proxy**

sample notes

**number of
decedents**

**questionnaire   coding information   bibliography
available   available**

links

availability of data

contacts

ADMINISTRATIVE INFORMATION

dataset   Medicare Claims   **abbrev** Medicare

parent study

first year   **last year**   1999

sponsor   Health Care Financing Administration

collector   Westat   **PI**

purpose   to track billing for health care services provided under the Medicare benefit to those eligible by age (65 years or older), disability, or end stage renal disease

topics   age, gender, race, geographic region, utilization to include hospitalizations, hospice, services, stays in skilled nursing facilities, outpatient, physician, and home health visits

design   continuous

baseline

followup

design notes

sample   41 million in 1998   **% proxy**

sample notes

number of   approximately 1,700 decedents per year
decedents

questionnaire   **coding information**   **bibliography**
available   **available**

links   linked to Social Security Administration records for pur-
                      poses of capturing decedents

availability of   Medicare Continous History File is available on 5% of
data   beneficiaries each year

contacts

ADMINISTRATIVE INFORMATION

dataset   Medicare Current Beneficiary Survey   **abbrev** MCBS

parent study   Medicare Claims

first year   1991   **last year**   1998

sponsor   HCFA

collector   Westat   **PI**

purpose   determine expenditures and sources of payment for all
                      health care services used by Medicare beneficiaries (in-
                      cluding noncovered services) and to trace changes in
                      health status and spending over time

topics   use of health services, expenditures, insurance coverage,
                      sources of payment, health status and functioning, and a
                      variety of demographic and behavioral information, such
                      as income, assets, living arrangements, family supports,
                      and access to medical care

design	four-year rotating panel
baseline	6,000 new beneficiaires are added each year
followup	interviewed every four months
design notes	originally not a rotating panel, but problems with follow up
sample	12,000 **% proxy**
sample notes	107 primary geographic sampling units, with oversampling in areas with high growth in population of elders
number of decedents	700 per year
questionnaire available	**coding information available** **bibliography**
links	Medicare claims and administrative data (in turn linked to Social Security Administration)
availability of data	purchased through HCFA
contacts	Director, Enterprises Databases Group, Office of Information and Systems, HCFA, 7500 Security Boulevard, Baltimore, MD 21244-1850; 410-786-3690

ADMINISTRATIVE INFORMATION

dataset	National Long Term Care Survey **abbrev** NLTCS
parent study	companion to the National Long-Term Care Channeling Demonstration (DHHS)
first year	1982 **last year** 1999
sponsor	Office of the Assistant Secretary for Planning and Evaluation (ASPE)
collector **PI**	Census administered; Duke University Kenneth Manton
purpose	to learn more about health, functioning, and social and economic factors among community-based disabled. The purpose of the Next of Kin Survey on decedents is to estimate the total long-term care costs and the extent of spend-down to qualify for Medicaid

topics	prevalence and patterns of functional limitations, both physical and cognitive; medical conditions and recent medical problems; use of health care services; kinds and amounts of formal and informal long-term care services used; demographic characteristics; public and private expenditures for health care services; and housing and neighborhood characteristics
design	list-based, longitudinal, panel design
baseline	In 1982, a random sample of 35,008 Medicare-eligible people >65 yr were screened for disability, yielding 6,393 chronically disabled community residents who qualified for in-person interviews. 1,925 interviews were completed with informal caregivers of disabled elders (of 2,349 identified)
followup	In 1984, all survivors were contacted to be reinterviewed. In addition, a sample of community residents who were not disabled in 1982 was added and a new sample of people who reached 65 years of age between 1982 and 1984 was added. This process was repeated in 1989, 1994, and 1999
design notes	Overall response rates ranged from 97.1% in 1982 to 95.4% in 1989; informal care supplement in 1982, 1989, 1999; next of kin decedents 1994; nursing home resident follow-back 1989; nutritional status 1994

sample	36,000	**% proxy**	23% 1984; 20% 1989

sample notes	55,000 screen interviews; 21,000 community detailed interviews, and 5,000 detailed institutional interviews in total for the 1982-1993 surveys; 1982: Medicare HISKEW file stratified geographically into LTC Primary Sampling Units, which were grouped into 173 long term care strata; one LTC PSU selected from each stratum
number of decedents	17,000 deaths identified from Medicare admin records (1982-1996): Next of Kin Supplement
questionnaire available	**coding information** **bibliography** **available**
links	linked to Medicare Part A and B most years; Medicare mortality records

availability of public use files available from Duke University
data   (http://cds.duke.edu)

contacts   Richard Suzman at NIA; William Marton at DALTCPT
                      (wmarton@osaspe.dhhs.gov)

ADMINISTRATIVE INFORMATION

dataset   National Health and Nutrition Examination   **abbrev**
                     NHFES

parent study   NHANES I

first year   1971   **last year**   1992

sponsor   NCHS/NIA

collector   **PI**

purpose   to investigate the association between factors measured
                     at baseline and the development of specific health condi-
                     tions. The three major objects are to study morbidity and
                     mortality associated with suspected risk factors, changes
                     over time in participant characteristics, and the natural
                     history of chronic disease and functional impairments

topics   self-reported medical conditions, activities of daily liv-
                     ing, health and nutrition habits and weight, physical ex-
                     aminations, laboratory tests, facility medical records,
                     death certificates

design   longitudinal follow up to a multistage, stratified sample

baseline   NHANES I data (1971-1975) included subsample that re-
                     ceived detailed study and an augmentation survey 1974-
                     1975.

followup   In 1982-1984, interviews were conducted with subject or
                     proxy for 84.8% of the eligible 14,407 cohort (11,361 alive,
                     2,022 deceased, 1,024 not traced); in 1986, those over 55
                     years old ($n = 3,980$) included 3,132 alive, 635 dead, and
                     213 not traced. In 1987, all ages cohort = 11,750 with
                     10,463 alive, 555 dead, and 732 not traced. In 1992, $n =$
                     11,195, with 8,687 still alive, 1,392 dead, 1,116 not traced.
                     Interviews in 1982-1984 were conducted in person; re-
                     maining years by phone with no physical assessment

design notes	four follow up waves: 1982, 1986, 1987, and 1992

sample	14,407	% proxy	1982-1984: 7.4%

sample notes 12,220 (84.8%) interviewed (or 91.3% of those traced); the NHANES I adults (25-74)   civilian noninstitutionalized population who completed a medical examination; included oversampling of persons living in poverty areas, women of childbearing age, and elderly (65+); a subsample of 6,913 were examined in greater depth and asked additional questions; an augmentation survey was conducted in 1974-1975

number of decedents 4,604 decedents: death certificates for 98%; interviews in 1992 with 1,130 (81.2%) of 1,392 decedents

questionnaire available **coding information available** **bibliography**

links a study ID number links any NHANES files

availability of data Mortality Data tape includes death certificate info on all decedents

contacts

ADMINISTRATIVE INFORMATION

dataset	National Health Interview Survey	abbrev NHIS

parent study

first year	1957	last year	2000

sponsor	NCHS

collector	U.S. Bureau of the Census	PI

purpose to produce statistics on disease, injury, impairment, disability, and related health topics on a uniform basis for the nation

topics

design cross sectional (area based household survey)

baseline About 40,000 households are interviewed in person each year (800 representative households selected each week to avoid seasonal bias), representing over 100,000 people

Responsible adult interviewed and asked about household members; core set of questions plus varying supplemental questions

followup

design notes   substantially redesigned in 1997; changes to capture outpatient surgery, services provided by other than MD providers; mental health services; improvements in measuring health status; symptoms instead of naming conditions; family-level data

sample   100,000 each year   **% proxy**

sample notes   area-based households; U.S. civilian, noninstitutionalized population; response rates 94.9% to 96.7%; coordinated with other Census surveys to avoid double survey of same household; Westat, Inc., studied sampling options for 1995 redesign

number of   32,431 decedents 1986-1994 (10,407 died within two years
decedents   of interview); linked to National Death Index

questionnaire   coding information   bibliography
available   available

links   National Death Index system beginning survey year 1986; vital status known through 1997

availability of Public use files on NCHS Website
data

contacts

ADMINISTRATIVE INFORMATION

dataset   Asset and Health Dynamics of the Oldest Old

abbrev   AHEAD

parent study

first year   1993   **last year**

sponsor

collector   **PI**

purpose   to provide an understanding of the implications of health dynamics in old age for transtitions in economic well-being, changes in family and martial status, and for reliance on public and private support systems

topics   demographic info; health, cognition, family structure and transfers, use and cost of health services, job status, income, net worth, subjective expectations, and insurance; these included physical tasks and personal care activities

design

baseline   Wave 1 conducted in 1993; response rate of 80%; those 70-79 were generally interviewed by telephone; those 80+ were generally interviewed in person

followup   Wave 2 took place in 1995 and 1996; reinterview rate of 95%; combined HRS/AHEAD in 1998

design notes

sample   8,222   % **proxy** avg 10.4% (increases with age; more men)

sample notes   initially noninstitutionalized persons born in 1923 or earlier (aged 70 years or older); Wave 1 = 8,222 respondents (and spouses). Wave 2 interviews were conducted with 7,039 of the 8,222 Wave I respondents and approximately 775 exit interviews with next of kin; multistage sample plan, with oversampling of Blacks, Hispanics, and Florida residents; dual sampliing frame using 81 of the 93 PSUs in HRS, then deleting half and replacing with selections from the HCFA-EDB file; compared to census files, the sample reflected population except for females aged 80 and over (more likely to be in nursing homes)

number of   775 from Wave 1
decedents

questionnaire   **coding information**   **bibliography**
available   **available**

links   Medicare (80% gave permission); Medicaid (fewer gave permission)

availability of data

contacts

Appendix B

Information on Selected Variables

INFORMATION ON SELECTED VARIABLES

dataset:	**LSOA**
site of death:	
cause of death:	
demographics:	SES
household:	household composition (age, relationship)
social supports:	social history
illnesses:	list of 13 serious conditions
physical symptoms:	
physical function:	6 ADLS, 6 IADLs, mobility, falling, dizziness, incontinence
psychological symptoms:	
quality of life:	
cognition:	
health services utilization support services:	
satisfaction with care:	

family care: helpers with key activities

out-of-pocket costs:

INFORMATION ON SELECTED VARIABLES

dataset: **NMFS**

site of death: cause of death:

demographics: SES

household: relationship of people living with

social supports:

illnesses: hypertension, heart attack, angina, stroke,
                                Alzheimer, dementia, mental health, diabetes,
                                cancer, asthma, emphysema, bronchitis,
                                cirrhosis, arthritis

physical symptoms:

physical function: mobility, ADL, IADL

psychological symptoms:

quality of life:

cognition: trouble understanding, remembering, recog-
                                nizing, problem behaviors

health services utilization support services:

satisfaction with care:

family care: did family members help/live with/help pay
                                for care

out-of-pocket costs: decedent funds and family expenses includes
                                "help at home"

INFORMATION ON SELECTED VARIABLES

dataset: **NHANES**

site of death: cause of death:

demographics: SES

household: delineates all members of household

social supports:

illnesses: extensive list of conditions

physical symptoms: extensive pain questionnaire

physical function: difficulty doing 19 activities

psychological symptoms:

quality of life:

cognition: self reported memory problems or confusion

health services utilization support services:

satisfaction with care:

family care:

out-of-pocket costs:

INFORMATION ON SELECTED VARIABLES

dataset: **MEPS**

site of death: cause of death:

demographics: SES

household:

social supports:

illnesses: respondent lists conditions for each family
                                    member

physical symptoms: pain

physical function: ADL, IADL, mobility questions

psychological symptoms: feeling anxious or blue

quality of life:

cognition: memory loss, confusion, decision making,
                                    supervision for safety

health services utilization support services:

satisfaction with care: general satisfaction, experience any diffi-
                                    culty, delay or lack of care

family care: detail info about caregivers

out-of-pocket costs: purchased medicines; alternative care (total
                                      expenditures only)

INFORMATION ON SELECTED VARIABLES

dataset: **MDS**

site of death: cause of death:

demographics: SES

household: marital status; lived alone prior to adm

social supports: family involvement; contact with relatives
                                  and close friends

illnesses: checklist plus open ICD coding

physical symptoms: pain, shortness of breath

physical function: ADLS specificially and pattern

psychological symptoms: mood, psychological well-being

quality of life:

cognition: memory, skills, delirium

health services utilization support services:

satisfaction with care:

family care:

out-of-pocket costs:

INFORMATION ON SELECTED VARIABLES

dataset: **PSID**

site of death: cause of death:

demographics: SES

household: relationships

social supports:

illnesses:

physical symptoms:

physical function: basic needs like dressing, bathing , eating

psychological symptoms:

quality of life:

cognition:

health services utilization support services:

satisfaction with care:

family care:

out-of-pocket costs: incl paid paid nurse/aide coming to home

INFORMATION ON SELECTED VARIABLES

dataset: **OASIS**

site of death: cause of death:

demographics: SES

household: spouse, other family, friend, paid help

social supports:

illnesses: diagnostic codes

physical symptoms: pain, shortness of breath, nausea, bowel
                                  function

physical function: ADLS, IADS

psychological symptoms: "emotional" problems

quality of life:

cognition: alter, requires prompting, requires assistance,
                                  confused

health services utilization support services:

satisfaction with care:

family care: who is caring, what types of assistance

out-of-pocket costs:

INFORMATION ON SELECTED VARIABLES

dataset: **NDI**

site of death: cause of death:

demographics: SES

household:

social supports:

illnesses:

physical symptoms:

physical function:

psychological symptoms:

quality of life:

cognition:

health services utilization support services:

satisfaction with care:

family car :

out-of-pocket costs:

INFORMATION ON SELECTED VARIABLES

dataset: **NHHCS**

site of death: cause of death:

demographics: SES

household: family, nonfamily

social supports:

illnesses: primary or other diagnoses

physical symptoms:

physical function: receives help from this agency regarding
                                   ADLs, IADLs

psychological symptoms:

quality of life:

cognition:

health services utilization support services:

satisfaction with care:

family care: relationship to primary caregiver

out-of-pocket costs: only as primary or secondary source of
                                payment

INFORMATION ON SELECTED VARIABLES

dataset: **NNHS**

site of death: cause of death:

demographics: SES

household: before adm to facility

social supports:

illnesses: primary and "other" diagnoses

physical symptoms:

physical function: ADLs, limited IALDs

psychological symptoms:

quality of life:

cognition:

health services utilization support services:

satisfaction with care:

family care:

out-of-pocket costs:

INFORMATION ON SELECTED VARIABLES

dataset: **MCBS**

site of death: cause of death:

demographics: SES

household: persons staying in the household social supports:

illnesses: long list

physical symptoms:

physical function: 6 ADLs, 6 IADLs

psychological symptoms:

quality of life:

cognition: memory, making decisions, concentrating

health services utilization support services:

satisfaction with care: general satisfaction, availability, convenience, information received, costs, etc.

family care :   who helps with ADLs/IADLs

out-of-pocket costs: equipment, prescriptions, alterations to house

INFORMATION ON SELECTED VARIABLES

dataset: **NHIS**

site of death: cause of death:

demographics: SES

household: relationships among all in household

social supports:

illnesses: "have you ever been told" broad domains: cardiovascular disease, respiratory conditions, etc.

physical symptoms: fatigue, tiredness, pain

physical function: single item about "major activity limitation"; ADLs, IADLs, Nagi

psychological symptoms: depression, anxiety, emotional problem

quality of life:

cognition: limited by difficulty remembering or confusions health services utilization support services:

satisfaction with care:

family care:

out-of-pocket costs: how much spent for medical care (exc hlth
                                    insurance, over counter

INFORMATION ON SELECTED VARIABLES

dataset: **NHEFS**

site of death: cause of death:

demographics: SES

household: # in household

social supports:

illnesses: ever had; doctor ever told arthritis, heart
                                    attack, stroke, diabetes, cancer, fx hip, os-
                                    teoporosis, etc.

physical symptoms: just arthritis (swelling, stiffness, pain)

physical function: Katz ADL; Rosow-Breslau, and Fries Func-
                                    tional

psychological symptoms:

quality of life:

cognition:

health services utilization support services:

satisfaction with care:

family care:

out-of-pocket costs:

INFORMATION ON SELECTED VARIABLES

dataset: **Medicare**

site of death: cause of death:

demographics: SES

household:

social supports:

illnesses: only as inferred from diagnostic codes on visits and stays

physical symptoms:

physical function:

psychological symptoms:

quality of life:

cognition:

health services utilization support services:

satisfaction with care:

family care:

out-of-pocket costs:

INFORMATION ON SELECTED VARIABLES

dataset: **NLTCS**

site of death: cause of death:

demographics: SES

household: identification of caregiver

social supports: how many times did see/talk with friends

illnesses: does . . . now have [30] conditions

physical symptoms:

physical function: 6 ADLs; 7 IADLs; Nagi items on range of motion and impairment; activity list

psychological symptoms: confusion or emotional problem

quality of life:

cognition: mini mental

health services utilization support services:

satisfaction with care:

family care: many details about who helps with ADLs and IADLs

out-of-pocket costs: who pays for help with ADLs/IADLs; payment for nursing home, homecare

INFORMATION ON SELECTED VARIABLES

dataset: **AHEAD**

site of death: cause of death:

demographics: SES

household: spouse, children, other

social supports: asked in HRS 1994 module

illnesses: major illnesses; severity reflected in type and intensity of care

physical symptoms: pain, shortness of breath, fatigue

physical function: difficulty with 12 physical tasks; if + then asked difficulty with 6 personal care activities

psychological symptoms: CESD used in HRS 1994

quality of life: 14 questions on AHEAD Wave 1

cognition: dementia screening instrument, memory, reasoning

health services utilization support services:

satisfaction with care:

family care :   living with, assisting ADLS

out-of-pocket costs: nursing home, prescriptions, in-home medical care, assistance with ADLs and IADLS

Appendix C

Workshop Agenda and Participants

Describing Death in America: What We Need to Know
WORKSHOP AGENDA
October 10, 2001

12:00 noon   INFORMAL LUNCH

1:00 pm   Welcome and introductions
      Thomas J. Smith, M.D., F.A.C.P., Workshop Chairman

1:15   Summary and status report on background paper
      June Lunney, Ph.D.

1:30   Remarks by individual workshop participants: Issues with existing data and suggestions for change

3:15   BREAK

3:30   Group discussion of recommendations to be considered by IOM

4:45   Wrap up
      Dr. Smith, Marilyn J. Field, Ph.D., Hellen Gelband

5:00   ADJOURN

Location: 1055 Thomas Jefferson Street, N.W.—"The Foundry"
Room 2004
Washington, D.C.

Describing Death in America
WORKSHOP PARTICIPANTS
October 10, 2001

Thomas J. Smith, M.D., F.A.C.P., *chair*
Medical College of Virginia at Virginia Commonwealth University

Amy B. Bernstein, Sc.D.
National Center for Health Statistics

Dwight Brock, Ph.D.
National Institute on Aging

Molla Sloane Donaldson, Dr.P.H.
National Cancer Institute

Vicki A. Freedman, Ph.D.
Polisher Institute, Philadelphia

Rosemary Gibson
The Robert Wood Johnson Foundation

Barbara Haupt, D.V.M.
National Center for Health Statistics

Marcia Levetown, M.D.
University of Texas

June Lunney, Ph.D.
Center to Improve Care of the Dying, The RAND Corporation

Timothy J. Moynihan, M.D.
Mayo Clinic—Medical Oncology

Peggy Parks
Center for Medicare and Medicaid Services

Phil Renner, M.B.A.
National Committee for Quality Assurance

Harry M. Rosenberg, Ph.D.
National Center for Health Statistics

Paul Schyve, M.D.
Joint Commission on Accreditation of Healthcare Organizations

Sidney M. Stahl, Ph.D.
National Institute on Aging

Joan Teno, M.D.
Brown University

Claudette Varricchio DSN, RN, FAAN
National Cancer Institute

Beth Virnig, Ph.D., M.P.H.
University of Minnesota